ELITENESS

How to Uncover Your Hidden Potential to Become an Elite Athlete in 9 Simple Steps!

DR. AUSTIN COHEN

Printed in the United States of America
Author: Austin Cohen
ISBN: 978-1-523-97892-2

TABLE OF CONTENTS

CHAPTER SIX 75-90

MINDSET

Step 7: Hour of Power
- How To Create a Positive Morning Routine
- Be Mindful As Well As Physical
- Section Takeaway

Step 8: Seeing Is Really Believing
- The Art of Visualization
- Proven Visualization Techniques
- Section Takeaway

Step 9: Getting Maximum Sleep
- What The Pros Say
- Tips To Get More Sleep!
- Section Takeaway

DEDICATION

This book is dedicated to the three people who have been a huge support for me and are no longer with us today. Poppy, Uncle Paul, and Poppa, thank you for all of the nuggets you have shared with me during your time on this Earth and know you are never forgotten.

ACKNOWLEDGEMENTS

There are many people I'd like to thank because none of this would be possible without their help or support.

First and foremost I must thank my amazing wife, Shira, for supporting me on all of my dreams and goals since the very first day we met. My vision and aspirations have always been enormous and your support has allowed me to achieve everything so far, which is why all of this success is owed to you. You have been not only the best wife—but an even better mother for taking care of our daughter to allow me to finish this book while still working full-time, training for an Ironman, and the millions of other projects I've had going on during the writing. Thank you.

My parents who have always stood by my side and who have made me the person I am today. My character, behavior, and discipline all come from you and I am forever grateful for how you raised me and brought me into this World.

My brother Michael and sister Shelby, you are my two best friends and thank you for always being honest with me about my character. Your love and support has given me guidance when writing this book and I am forever grateful for our relationships.

Emily Bridgers, there is so much I could say but honestly you have been one of the most amazing people I have ever met. Your humbleness, spirit, and support since 2014 has been inspiring and I will always be grateful that we connected. Thanks for putting together such a beautiful foreword and for helping me with this book no matter how successful and busy you have become. I will always be here for you too—thank you from the bottom of my heart.

Thanks also goes to my office staff for all of the time they spent looking at my old articles and being honest with me during the early stages of this book. The commitment you have to my practice has allowed me such freedom to get this book to the public and I hope all of you know how grateful I am for each and every one of you.

Stacie Tovar, Gordon Beckham and Dolvett Quince, thanks for trusting me with your healthcare needs and sharing your stories in this book for everyone to read and be inspired by. The three of you are superb athletes from different walks of life and have so much to share with people about your amazing successes.

And lastly, thank you to my editor Kerrie Lee Brown—you have taken my manuscript and transformed it into a readable book for the general public that I am very proud of. I am grateful that I found you as your guidance has helped me with the flow of my content; and you've shaped it in a way that makes sense for my readers to see my vision in creating The Eliteness Movement.

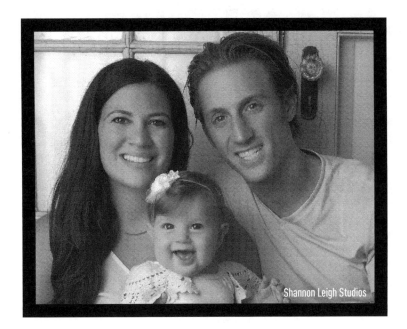

Shannon Leigh Studios

FOREWORD

I had the pleasure of meeting Dr. Cohen back in 2012 when he signed up to take my adult gymnastics class that I coached once a week with a group of CrossFit athletes. He was the only male in my class, but that didn't seem to faze him.

Over the weeks it became clear that he was in my class to expand his knowledge of movement, strength and flexibility for his own athletic endeavors—and it wasn't long before he was proficient in certain gymnastics moves, which helped him become a better athlete. I was impressed by his dedication.

Although this particular class was held fairly late at night—it became obvious to me that Dr. Cohen was on a mission as he came to class every week with tons of energy and was always eager to learn. However, some weeks he would have to miss class due to speaking engagements or travel, and that's when I learned that he was very successful in his career as a chiropractor.

About a year later, I ran into Dr. Cohen at a local CrossFit competition. He had been following my CrossFit journey for the past three years and knew that I had fallen just short of my goal of making the CrossFit Games three years in a row.

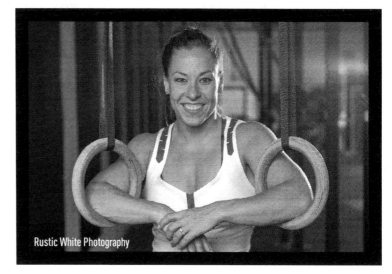

Rustic White Photography

It was then that he told me he could get me to the next level!

With the same positive and eager attitude, Dr. Cohen convinced me to set up a chiropractic appointment in his office the next week. Fast-forward two years later, and I seriously have not missed one week of adjustments since. Dr. Cohen has definitely been able to help me take my athletic career to the next level. He was certainly true to his word. With Dr. Cohen's help I have remained injury-free and achieved quite a few athletic and personal goals.

In 2014, I finally qualified for the CrossFit Games and went on to become the 6th fittest female in the world.

In 2015, a high point in my life was representing Team USA in the CrossFit Invitational where our team came out on top over Australia, Canada, and Europe. I also had a few other significant finishes in competitions throughout the year. I worked extremely hard to push myself physically and mentally to reach my athletic potential—and in doing so, inspired many people along the way.

Also in 2015, I remained injury-free and qualified for the CrossFit Games for the second year in a row!

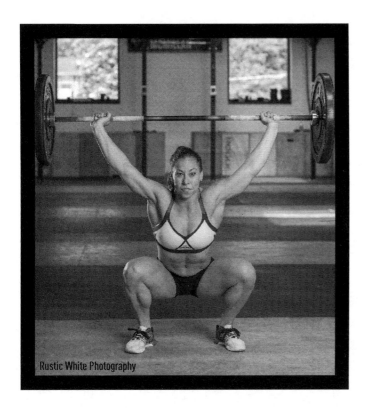

Rustic White Photography

During my journey and still today, Dr. Cohen has not only been there for chiropractic care, but is constantly sharing his advice to becoming my best self. He has provided nutrition advice, recovery tips for outside of the office, traveled to my competitions, offered business and financial strategies, and is always researching the next best tool to help me achieve my goals. In fact, Dr. Cohen goes out of his way to help all of his clients in the same way he has helped me, while still remaining committed to living the same kind of lifestyle himself.

This book breaks down many of the ways you can tap into your hidden potential and never plateau in life. It has helped me a great deal and I am very grateful for Dr. Cohen's program. Here's what you can look forward to in this book:

In this book, Dr. Cohen hones in on your nutrition and supplements, which can be a make or break acumen for those looking to get to the next level. There are certain foods and minerals that the body needs as fuel and Dr. Cohen does a great job simplifying that process while being direct and to the point about what is needed to reach your goals.

Dr. Cohen also looks at the most common reasons why someone gets hurt or is limited in movements and creates unique systems and tools to help move their progress forward. I use his dynamic stretches on a regular basis before and after competitions and they have helped me tremendously with maxing out my performance.

And in conclusion, Dr. Cohen shares his insight on the importance of mental training and visualization—the mental aptitude of eliteness—and what it takes to think like a professional. He also provides a few case studies of athletes he's trained in various sports. All of the sections in this book give you a good sense of the missing elements you need to discover in order to become your best self—which are usually the blind spots people don't think of to becoming elite.

With all this being said, I personally challenge you to define what eliteness means in your life and use this book to provide you with the best steps to become more elite in all aspects of your life. It worked for me and I am still learning and reaching my goals.

Emily Bridgers
CrossFit Athlete/Owner of CrossFit Terminus
Atlanta, Georgia

PREFACE

WHY I WROTE THIS BOOK

When I was 13 years old, something critical happened that would change my life forever. I found myself mowing my parents' lawn during summer break with my shirt off, and out of nowhere my neighbor yelled; "Put the bird in the cage!"

I was really confused. At such a young, impressionable age, all I could fathom was that possibly she was talking about our pet finch or some wild bird she saw flying around the house… But I was wrong. Turns out she was talking about my scrawny bird chest. I still remember that moment like it was yesterday, and ever since that time I have been determined to find a way to build muscle mass.

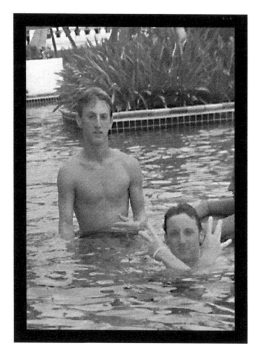

Call me crazy, but it's become my life-long mission to help others with similar experiences too.

However the challenge I faced at the time was:

1. Commitment

2. Self-discipline

This scenario played on my mind for a long time—and I was determined to change my physique. It's terribly sad and disheartening that these types of experiences we have as children can shape our thoughts, feelings and confidence as we grow up. But I was determined to change for me, not for them, and prove that my experience while helping my parents with their yard work would help me become a strong individual inside and out.

So I made a commitment to myself to start making healthy lifestyle choices, even in my teens, throughout my young adult life. I tried several strategies including: biking, isolated strength training (typical machines found at a gym), boutique gyms, etc.

During my trials and tribulations and experimentation, I ultimately found what kind of forms of physical activity worked for me and what did not. I ended up losing interest and getting discouraged several times because I didn't see the results I thought I was on track to. Life started to get in the way and I soon realized that when we are not invested in what we are doing 100 percent—we will never reach our desired outcome.

So I decided to come up with a plan to help others reach their goals—while I was still searching for the answer to my own fitness issues. In doing so, I learned to observe others and I saw some of my skinny friends go from scrawny to brawny in a few months. Their secret was supplementation with artificial substances (i.e. steroids, artificially-caffeinated pre-workout supplements, and protein powders with chemical additives). Sure, this mantra can be a quick fix to creating gains in muscle, but there can be serious consequences long-term on one's health when using these kinds of substances. Of my friends who put on muscle mass the right (and healthy) way, each one of them gave the same advice to get the best results: commitment and self-discipline coupled with proper diet and functional fitness.

I was convinced! Becoming a committed person no matter what life threw at me was the only way I was going to get where I needed to go in my goals.

In 2006, I decided to challenge myself beyond what I thought was possible and I committed to run the Chicago Marathon. I knew I would have to push myself to train for this race because my longest distance to that date had only been 6.2 miles (which is 20 miles fewer than a full marathon).

I CERTAINLY HAD MY WORK CUT OUT FOR ME.

For 16 weeks, I followed a running regimen that prepared me to accomplish all 26.2 miles. I even trained late at night when I got home from my chiropractic classes after a long day. My runs still got accomplished because 1) I committed to myself, and 2) I knew that if I didn't train, I would get hurt. These were the biggest motivating factors for me.

I EMOTIONALLY CROSSED THE FINISH LINE OF THE **CHICAGO MARATHON** WITH A TIME OF 3 HOURS AND 53 MINUTES. WHEN MY RUNS MAXED OUT AT 6 MILES, I STILL NEVER THOUGHT I WOULD FINISH ANOTHER 20 ON TOP OF THAT. **BUT I DID.**

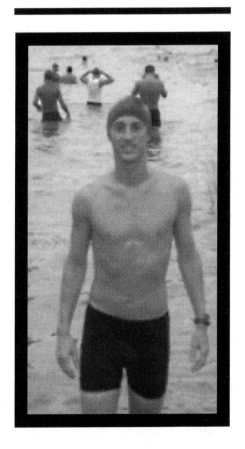

On October 22, 2006, I emotionally crossed the finish line of the Chicago Marathon with a time of 3 hours and 53 minutes. When my runs maxed out at 6 miles, I still never thought I would finish another 20 on top of that. But I did.

Accomplishing this marathon proved to me I could set high goals and accomplish them, no matter how far-fetched or beyond my limits it sounded at the time.

Commitment is addictive. Between 2006 and 2009, I completed one more marathon, one sprint triathlon, and one Olympic triathlon. Training for these high-caliber races changed me forever.

Hard work and dedication became second nature to me and staying committed to a goal created strong habits inside me that also carried into other areas of my life.

Then, at some point in the midst of finishing these races, I lost track of my "why" for getting into fitness. I just wanted to build muscle mass and focus on the "how" so I could help others do the same.

In 2010, I recommitted to gaining muscle mass and knew it was going to be a different kind of discipline than what it took for the endurance training for marathons. Building the kind of muscle mass I envisioned for myself required higher levels of intensity, so I was going to have to turn myself into a machine in every aspect of life.

I WANTED TO BECOME AN ELITE ATHLETE!

To accomplish this new goal, I made three commitments:

1. Join a CrossFit™ gym.

2. Eat a strictly Paleo diet.

3. Hire a fitness coach to program my workouts.

Every Sunday, my fitness coach tailored five days of workouts for me, and I learned the benefits of eating according to the Paleo diet. This type of training really pushed my body each workout, and I definitely felt the soreness in my muscles the next day. I was getting stronger as each week passed, and I was finally reaching the goal I set way back when I was younger as a result of my neighbor calling me scrawny.

My journey of becoming a stronger and fitter athlete has changed me in more ways than one. In short, here are some of my personal statistics from 2010 to 2013:

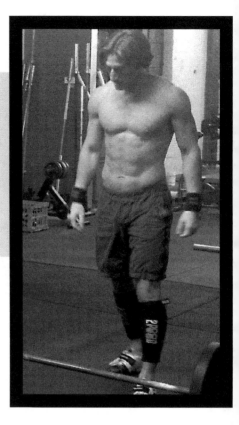

Weight Gain/Muscle Mass:

- 155 pounds to 190 pounds
- Body fat: 10% down to 5%
- Back Squat increased from 200 to 355
- Clean increased from 155 to 245
- Front squat increased from 235 to 330
- Fran (Thrusters and Pull-Ups, sets of 21-15-9) time decreased from 9:45 to 3:11

Committing to becoming a better (elite) athlete translated into something I never could have imagined. The benefits of faster workout times and increased lifts, muscle mass, and weight gain for me were exciting—but the most powerful gains of all were the non-tangibles, including a stronger relationship with my wife, increased self-confidence, and more tools to share with my patients on how they can improve their health as well.

Every day I think about a quote one of my mentors once told me:

"HOW YOU DO ANYTHING IN LIFE IS HOW YOU DO EVERYTHING IN LIFE."

I see this quote come to fruition every day in my chiropractic clinic when new patients get SO EXCITED about starting chiropractic care and changing their lifestyles.

However, it saddens me when some of them disappear from the schedule after two weeks. Looking back at the people's charts who do not keep up with their consultations, and trying to figure out what went wrong and why they may have felt the commitment factor was too much, I've realized these clients are usually the same people who join the gym in January and quit in February. Unfortunately there will always be people who cannot commit to relationships, and continuously go on and off diet plans. If you look in other areas of their lives, they also might have procrastination issues.

On the flip side, most of my clients are equally as excited about starting a corrective care program, and they come to appointments on time (and cancel ahead of time if they need to miss). They are enthusiastic about their progress in the office, and talk encouragingly about their body's potential to heal. They, too, are people who tend to have successful communication and relationships—and have consistent workout regimens they follow and who take initiative in creating and following through with plans.

Granted, the different types of traits in people I have described on the previous pages do not encompass every person; these are just the over-arching patterns I have seen at my chiropractic practice and within my professional circles. My goal is to reach anyone who wants to make improvement and see how far their physical and mental aspirations can take them. I am here to guide, advise and help you make decisions that will get you to a point where you feel you are beyond your normal self and able to reach an elite status within your fitness.

To conclude, I want each and every one of you to live a great life—and the key is to show up for what you are committing yourself to, and begin to realize the change you can make in yourself through hard work and escalating your efforts beyond 100 percent. And eventually you will see the ripple effect of your accomplishments on your relationships outside of the gym and chiropractic appointments—which is extremely motivating to others as well.

Let this book be a WAKE-UP call to you in an empowering way. My hope is that you realize your true potential in all that you can do in life. Eliteness provides *9 Simple Steps to Help You Become a Healthier Person and Better Athlete*—but more importantly, it will help you become your best self.

In Health,

Dr. Austin Cohen

Corrective Chiropractic, Atlanta, Georgia

P.S. HOW TO READ THIS BOOK—TIPS FOR EASIER READING!

Let me be honest and upfront with you from the beginning. Becoming elite is hard work—but it's worth it! This book has A LOT of useful information to reach your goals so don't let the number of pages intimidate you. When I decided to write this book I knew right off the bat that I wanted to help people reach their potential. And since I am a very upfront and bullet-point-type-of-guy, I knew that my book would reflect this demeanor as well. Let me assure you— there is no fluff in this book.

In order for you to grasp everything I have included on these pages, I have included Section Takeaways after every "Step" as helpful 'mini guides'. They will help streamline the important points for you. My hope is that you will use the Section Takeaways and designated Notes pages at the end of the chapters as your personal eliteness log and/or an area you can write down the gems you need to make changes. You may want to tear out these pages and throw them in your gym bag as well so they're always close to you.

I find it very interesting that every time I do a speech I have people come up to me and tell me how motivated they are to follow my advice and lead a healthier life. But often when I check in with them months down the road, they haven't taken the necessary steps to get there. Don't be one of those people! I want you to take the next step. I've given you the opportunity to become your BEST SELF with all of the top-notch information you need to lead a better life. So use the Notes pages to jot down what you need to remember and keep them close to you at all times.

My goal and hope is that you read this book and find value—but that you also TAKE ACTION and begin to make change. The only way that will happen is if you follow each step and retain the information in bite-sized pieces.

INTRODUCTION
OVERVIEW

WHAT IS ELITENESS?

Eliteness is about taking your body from where it is now—physically and mentally—and maximizing it in order to meet its potential. The purpose of this book, appropriately named Eliteness, is not to make every person a professional athlete (unless that is your goal) but rather to help people meet their own expectations and do what is necessary to become their best athlete and ultimately their best self. Most people innately have a perception of what it looks like to "live up to their potential" but what if there was a way to reach even further? What is there was a secret formula that could help maximize your expectations to meet your ultimate goals personally and professionally? What if there was a program based and emerging industry movement in which you could push your physical and mental limits to the max and break down barriers all in the name of reaching "eliteness"?

In other words, eliteness is the act of breaking through your barriers and moving beyond the capacity you think you are capable of achieving. Eliteness is not a hierarchy or status but more about taking what the 1 percent of athletes do in their journey to becoming elite and integrating it into your life—the every day.

Many of us have regular 9 to 5 jobs so we need simple strategies to becoming elite and living the "eliteness" lifestyle and if you follow these unique strategies outlined in this book you will do just that.

WHAT IS AN ELITE ATHLETE?

An elite athlete is someone who consistently ranks in the top 1 percent of everything they do athletically. Many times these over-achievers may get paid professionally but many times they can be the average person too. Eliteness is a "9 Step Process to Uncovering Your Potentials" to becoming elite, which is the greatest version of you.

This book may not ever make you a professional athlete but if you are breaking through your own barriers, reaching new capacities (new heights!), and achieving the goals you set for yourself, then you are living the eliteness ideal.

WHO SHOULD READ THIS BOOK?

This book is aimed at people who strive to be better then they are today. In particular, this program is designed with many CrossFit athletes in mind—those who already know the benefits of pushing the boundaries in the gym and their nutrition on a daily basis. But you don't have to aspire to become a professional athlete—you just have to be looking for something beyond the ordinary in your health and fitness life.

Most people were not born with a "pro" gene but that doesn't mean you can't reach for the highest potential possible to perform at an elite level to lead overall healthier lives. You can do that by incorporating the 9 protocols in this book. Good luck!

CHAPTER ONE

WHY YOU SHOULD JOIN "THE ELITENESS MOVEMENT"

What I find very interesting is how our society is still quick to make judgments of others. We live in a culture where the majority of people question or are closed off to new ideas, and they often dismiss new methodologies without finding out more.

The truth is that a lot of people are afraid to try new things—because they don't know what the outcome will be, or because it takes hard work to even see an outcome. It's the fear of the unknown.

I am hoping by reading this book you will see that opening your mind to new ways of doing things will not only help you in the long run (particularly where your health, fitness and longevity are concerned) but by figuring out where your thoughts and ideas can lead you to being your best self.

There have been numerous studies conducted at high-caliber schools and institutions suggesting that living an unhealthy lifestyle and eating the wrong foods will lead you down a path of disease and health risks. For instance, research has been done on the effects of sedentary lifestyles and one of the most prominent researchers, Dr. James Levine, director of the Mayo Clinic-Arizona State University Obesity Solutions Initiative, is noted for saying: "Sitting is the new smoking".[1]

Dr. Levine suggests that more and more people are dying of diseases related to sitting. In fact according to this study, researchers proved the correlation between a sedentary lifestyle and two big killers diabetes and heart disease. Research has also been done numerous times on people with high inflammatory diets and their correlation to chronic disease.

---

[1]Wilmot EG, Edwardson CL, Achana FA, et al. *Sedentary time in adults and the association with diabetes, cardiovascular disease and death*: systematic review and meta-analysis. Diabetologia 2012;55:2895–905.

So what does this mean to you? In basic terms, it means that if you choose to follow an unhealthy lifestyle (and dismiss new ideas of how to strive and survive by focusing on being your best self) then these diseases may become a reality for you.

Does everyone who lives a sedentary life and eats high-inflammatory foods die of chronic disease? No, of course not! My grandmother-in-law ate like garbage and had an extremely sedentary life due to being in a wheelchair from spinal stenosis and lived to her late 90's. But the point is that there is research to support what I've said previously and the odds are much greater for people who are more sedentary and eat unhealthy food.

On the flip side, do people who move all day and eat anti-inflammatory foods live forever? Again the answer is No. However the difference is that those people are maximizing their genetic expression and drastically raising their chances of not becoming a victim to the chronic diseases.

The point to all of this is that heart disease, cancer, and diabetes could become reality for you. There are no guarantees. Eliteness offers a solution for you to change your ways and ultimately change your lifestyle options.

When I began living a proactive lifestyle of getting chiropractic adjustments regularly, maintenance massages, eating a Paleo diet, meditating, acupuncture, setting goals, and giving lectures it became obvious to me how many people said: "Are you in a cult" or "This lifestyle sounds so cultish". This may be because I chose to start following a strict regimen and would not steer from my healthy ways.

But personally I am not affected by what others think because what they don't realize is that this is a movement that a lot of elite athletes and weekend warriors who are serious about their health are implementing into their lives.

NUTRITION, EXERCISE AND POSITIVE THINKING ARE POWERFUL MECHANISMS TO HEALING THE BODY, AND THEY CREATE A TITANIUM INTERNAL ENVIRONMENT FOR YOUR BODY TO THRIVE.

As a health professional, I would rather you follow a lifestyle of eating healthy, working out, setting goals, and creating a better life for yourself. I did it and so can you. But you have to want it like I did. You have to want to change your lifestyle for the better and follow through with your commitment.

Unfortunately, society for the most part follows a lifestyle quite opposite to this—one of genetically modified food, sedentary lifestyles, negative thoughts, obsessions with reality television, and living a social life that exists primarily of technology over face-to-face interaction.

This my friends, is what I call a "cult" because most people are not aware of what they're doing to themselves on the day to day and as a result are hurting their health and social skills as a whole. This is my opinion but I know many who feel the same. I am here to help you unleash your potential by following an easy 9-step program to eliteness or greatness in your life.

Another example that proves my way of thinking is evident on the TV show "The Biggest Loser." Have you noticed how much dedication and commitment the contestants have who are trying to lose a lot of weight? No one gains weight during the season and for the most part his or her weight-loss goals are met. This takes a lot of determination and lifestyle changes. Every person on that show loses weight because they are very committed to working out and eating healthy.

Unfortunately it has become obvious that some of the contestants on this show suffer from what I call "Environmental Genetics" – meaning the environment they most likely grew up in was very unhealthy. They may have been subjected to lack of movement and mobility, poor nutrition choices, and negative thinking. For those who did suffer from a "Biological Genetic" challenge, they were able to overcome the turning on of those genes by changing their lifestyles. Nutrition, exercise and positive thinking are powerful mechanisms to healing the body, and they create a titanium internal environment for your body to thrive.

My observation is that society needs to change its way of thinking about nutrition, health and fitness, as well as positive thinking. The way to do this is to simply cut out the excuses and GET REAL! You only get ONE life on this Earth, ONE life to thrive, succeed, and fulfill your purpose. Don't waste it!

NOTES

CHAPTER TWO

NEVER PLATEAU IN LIFE AGAIN

When I was 24 years old, I remember a speaker at a seminar once saying "in our lives there is no peak and no final destination of success in any category: professional, health, relationships, or finance." This has stuck with me ever since because it's true! Our lives are like a seesaw where we are either moving up or moving down but never staying stagnant.

When you eat dinner, your body is either getting healthier or getting sick; when you show up to work you are either increasing your wealth or decreasing your wealth; and when you spend time with your significant other, your relationship is either getting stronger or weaker. There are no standstills!

Since the seminar, I have made it a mission to catch myself on a downward turn or plateau and move back up to experience an even greater life.

When I started doing CrossFit™ several years back I noticed I usually plateaued after certain Olympic lifts, and certain movements I was never improving no matter how much I practiced them. My times would stay consistent even though I would be in the top 20 percent of each class while never surpassing the better athletes. When I caught myself in these plateaus, I would say to myself "What can I do or who do I need to be in order to be in the top 5 percent?"

I was already getting chiropractic adjustments weekly and eating a strict Paleo diet at the time but I still wanted to know what could be done to get better. So I began to implement massage therapy into my regimen twice a month to help with soft tissue and this increased my gymnastic movements (flexibility).

A few months later, I went onto Kelly Starrett's blog called MobilityWOD® at MobilityWod.com (voted top 10 fitness blog in 2012) and began implementing his mobility work before workouts to reduce risk of injury. Kelly's unique approach to idealizing movement and fixing the underlying pathomechanics issues are now touted as the Starrett Method of Movement & Mobility. I also hired someone to design a specific training program for me to target these trouble spots and my weaknesses—which helped strengthen the muscles that needed work.

Eventually I noticed my times getting faster and my lifts improving.

As we move into the meat of this book and the program I personally develop for you to improve your desired results and reach your potential—I want you to think about how I too have been where you are today. Perhaps you've hit a plateau and your body is not responding to your usual workout, or maybe you're at a standstill with your regimen and need some guidance on how to change it up. That's why I've created this guide for you. This book does not need to be read from front-to-back as it is set up for you to go back-and-forth through the different chapters as often as you need to make advancements. I have outlined a variety of tips, tricks and strategies for you to reach your potential and change your life forever.

WHEN I CAUGHT MYSELF IN THESE PLATEAUS, I WOULD SAY TO MYSELF **"WHAT CAN I DO OR WHO DO I NEED TO BE IN ORDER TO BE IN THE TOP 5 PERCENT?"**

NOTES

CHAPTER THREE

INTRODUCTION TO THE 9 STEPS

The good news is that you've gotten this far and you haven't given up on learning how to reach your potential. The bad (or challenging news) is that you haven't even gotten to the part where we outline specifically what you have to do to attain your goals. But that's the exciting part!

You are now one chapter away from the meat and potatoes of this book but before moving forward I wanted to introduce you to each section. The sections are not listed in order of importance as each section has its equal share of the pie.

The sections are broken down into the following:
1. Nutrition
2. Mobility
3. Mindset

If you take these 3 concepts above and began working on each regularly and finding ways to incorporate them into your regimen—then your training and performance will automatically improve. Each of those sections will make an important impact on your performance and can help you tap into your potential.

But some of you (well, most of you, and this included me) need something more specific.

Most of us are already working out hard and performing at a high level, but we're not meeting our desired results. The problem is that most of us never realize how much more greatness (or eliteness) we could experience by utilizing certain steps.

That's why I have broken down the essentials for you over the next few chapters so you will have the latest strategies at your fingertips all the time.

NOTES

CHAPTER FOUR

NUTRITION

STEP 1: EVERY DAY EATING FOR ENHANCED PERFORMANCE

As we move into this next section on what you need to eat for optimal performance as an athlete, let me first share my three big no-no's:

❶ Grain + **❷** Pasteurized Dairy + **❸** Processed Sugar = **Body Destroyers**

As I've already mentioned, I am a huge advocate of the Paleo diet (hunter-gatherer) and I believe that everyone in our culture should implement this lifestyle. The reason I am such a big fan of this diet is because with the Paleo diet you are cutting out anything refined or processed that could lead to future degenerative diseases. It is a very nutritious way of eating—in fact research says it is how our ancestors used to eat and survive as hunters and gatherers.

It is my belief that if you want to perform your absolute best at the gym and in your own life, then eating clean with foods that work for you in a most natural state (not against you) will give you the greatest advantage.

In fact, in 2009 research was done that showed cholesterol for healthy individuals went down 16 percent, triglycerides went down 35 percent, and blood pressure dropped in those people who followed this lifestyle.[2]

In 2013, the Paleo diet became a household name again and is still one of the most popular diets. It continues to have an amazing impact on people all around the globe because it works and is known to be one of the healthiest plans.

By initially eliminating these three ingredients from your diet (grain, pasteurized dairy, and processed sugar) you will immediately begin to notice gains in your performance and overall weight-loss management. Most people see the positive effects within the first week or two.

[2] Frassetto, et al. Metabolic and Physiologic Improvements from Consuming a Paleolithic, Hunter-Gatherer type diet. European Journal of Clinical Nutrition, 2009.

Now many of you may say that taking out these food groups eliminates 90 percent of what you typically eat, and I agree with that statement. The average person eats cereal, toast, or a bagel for breakfast, a sandwich for lunch, and then pasta or pizza for dinner, followed by some sugary dessert. This all ties back to how the majority of society lives nowadays but as you know this is not healthy—and certainly not a way to make gains and reach your goals.

Put it this way, the reason you probably picked up this book or attended one of my seminars is because you strive to be an elite athlete. You want to be the best version of yourself, and status quo is not good enough. So let's break down exactly what you should eat throughout the day into timeframes to have a better understanding of how easy it is to eliminate the Big 3.

BREAKFAST

Eating protein first thing in the morning is essential for people who work out regularly, particularly at an intense level. Hence, protein and a certain amount of fat help maintain a stable blood sugar level, so you do not experience an energy spike or crash in the middle of the morning.

ORGANIC MEATS:

When it comes to eating meat (your best source of protein), it is important that you choose animals that have been pasture-raised and that haven't been fed any antibiotics, growth hormones, or genetically modified corn, grains, or soy products. Remember, whatever the animal eats or whatever gets injected into that animal goes directly into your body as you ingest the protein.

Clean meats are an excellent source of protein, high-quality fat and nutrients, so starting your day with a healthy portion is going to set your day on a positive trajectory. Some good breakfast meats are bacon, turkey bacon, sausage, or chicken-sausage.

PASTURE-RAISED EGGS:

Eggs tend to be a big 'go-to' for people who train because you can make a dozen hard-boiled eggs on Sunday and eat them throughout the week for breakfast. One of my favorite dishes is to mash up the hard boiled eggs with avocado to make a healthy egg salad—I not only get ample protein from the eggs, but the avocado also provides healthy fats and several powerful nutrients.

You can also make scrambled eggs with a few veggies in fewer than 10 minutes by heating up coconut oil or organic/grass-fed butter in a salute pan. Toss veggies into the pan, and salute for about 2 minutes. Then, add the scrambled eggs, and cook for 4-5 minutes. Voila!

FRUIT:

Fruit provides essential nutrients to the body as well, but I usually do not recommend eating fruit only for breakfast. Doing so can lead to a blood sugar spike, so make sure to pair your fruit choices with appropriate proteins and healthy fats.

PALEO CEREAL (USUALLY MADE WITH ALMOND FLOUR):

My favorite products are "noGRAINola" from Paleo Primal Concepts and Steve's Paleo Goods' "Cinnamon Paleo Cereal." These "cereals" are affordable, healthy, and great for the whole family.

Serve with almond, coconut, or hemp milk that does not have carrageenan on the ingredient list. Carrageenan is an agent used in products to increase thickness but when it hits the digestive system creates an inflammatory response. Veteran carrageenan researcher Joanne Tobacman, MD, said: "Carrageenan predictably causes inflammation, which can lead to ulcerations and bleeding".

For those who want to go to the next level, make your own fresh almond milk. It is super easy and tastes delicious!

Recipe ingredients:

1/2 cup raw, soaked almonds
1/4 cup raw, soaked hazelnuts
2 cups water
5 Medjool dates

Directions:

Blend all ingredients together.
Pour blended mix over cheesecloth into a big bowl.
Refrigerate, and enjoy!
(Use the scratch in the cheesecloth to make muffins.)

LUNCH & DINNER

SALADS

Many people who want to eat clean and healthy know that salad is going to be a big part of the regimen. Salads are simple and inexpensive to make, and they are a nutrient-dense punch to the body. If your goal is to put on muscle, add a healthy protein to your salad to keep loading up the body with BCAA's. As far as salad dressings, there are several websites and blogs that give great Paleo salad dressing recipes.

Here is a simple dressing I make at home that is nutrient-dense and tastes great:

Dr. Cohen's Salad Dressing

Add Together:

Extra Virgin Olive Oil

Bragg Apple Cider Vinegar

Oregano

Himalayan Sea Salt

Nutritional Yeast

BEEF/CHICKEN

As stated in the breakfast section, eating clean meats is non-negotiable for people looking to function and perform their best. Non-organic meats are typically abundant in inflammatory ingredients and wreak havoc on the body, especially on the digestive system. There are also extremely high levels of antibiotics and hormones in conventional meats, which take a toll on your body's ability to function at its optimum.

So while clean meats can sometimes be a bit more expensive, look at it as a long-term investment in yourself, as you will be less likely to spend copious amounts of money on future medical bills due to chronic diseases.

Some Tips:

Prepare a dozen pieces of baked or grilled chicken to eat throughout the week. Efficiency and advanced preparation are keys to sticking with a healthy meal plan each day. Make it a game and it won't seem like work! Find 52 different ways to season a chicken to make cooking a fun daily experience rather than a chore.

When it comes to preparing beef, I take grass-fed ground sirloin and put it in a pan with either ghee or coconut oil. Once slightly heated, I like to add a variety of different vegetables such as broccoli, red onion, red pepper, mushrooms, etc. This dish is best eaten at night because it is heavy and therefore your body can digest all of the nutrients while you are resting and recovering for the next day.

Sometimes people get stuck on the idea that their food has to look a certain way, or the recipes have to be a laundry list of different food items to be healthy, but remember simplicity is important. Athletes that want to make superb gains in their physique, or increase their level of fitness, eat for fuel and focus on filling their plates with high-density nutrients. An ideal meal is as easy as throwing meat into a pan with veggies! And only eat until you are full.

PIZZA

Yes, you read that correctly! The fact is ANYTHING can be made healthy as long as you choose the correct ingredients. There are so many Paleo resources that have tons of healthy takes on recipes—one of my favorite books is *Paleo Comfort Foods*. In fact if you Google "Paleo pizza recipes" you will find numerous healthy variations using alternatives to traditional breaded crusts like cauliflower or meat, topped with loads of vegetables. Yum!

SNACKS

BANANA/ALMOND BUTTER WRAP

When it comes to snacks, most people want fast, healthy and convenient. But they are not always easily available. I am an advocate for snacks so long as people make the right choices of what to eat. One of my all-time favorite snacks is a Paleo Wrap made by Julian Bakery as a base, spread with raw almond butter, banana slices, and toasted coconut flakes. It is super fast and extremely easy to make. These wraps can also be used for lunch or dinner items as an alternative to bread.

TRAIL MIX

The great thing about making your own trail mix is you can diversify it to your taste buds. You can bring this snack anywhere, but be sure to not get too carried away and eat too much trail mix in one sitting. While nutritious in appropriate amounts, too many nuts and seeds can be difficult on the digestive system and lead to excessive weight gain. Here is a list of suggested ingredients that are Paleo-approved to add into your trail mix:

Almonds (raw)

Cashews (raw)

Brazil Nuts (raw)

Shredded Coconut Flakes (no sugar added)

Pumpkin Seeds (raw)

Sunflower Seeds (raw)

Raisins (no sugar added)

Enjoy Life Chocolate Chips (dairy, soy, and nut free)

DR. COHEN'S TOP 3 PALEO/PRIMAL COMPANIES

There are several companies out there that make great, healthy snacks, and the more we support them, the more they will grow and prosper. As the popularity of eating Paleo/primal grows, the more companies will try to jump on the bandwagon. But with that being said, be extremely careful whom you trust because some companies sneak harmful ingredients into their products without consumers knowing.

Here are three companies that I recommend:

Pete's Paleo

Steve's Paleo Goods

Paleo Primal Concepts

DESSERT

Yes, you can eat healthy desserts on the Paleo diet!

The trick here is once again going online and doing some research for healthy alternatives to your favorite sweets. For example, if you love brownies, search "Paleo brownie recipes" to find a plethora of options and so on.

My favorite Paleo desserts are cheesecake and chocolate pudding. For the cheesecake, make sure to use cashew cheese (i.e. cashews that have been soaked and blended) as they create a great consistency and taste even better than the 'real cheesecake' that is filled with sugar and dairy.

There are countless Paleo chocolate pudding recipes online too. This dish usually includes avocado as a base, which may sound strange at first. But once you taste it—topped with whipped coconut milk on the top—you will never look back. Be sure to also use Fair Trade chocolate when making the recipe. Chocolate pudding has even become a favorite amongst my nieces and daughter!

SECTION TAKEAWAY: EVERY DAY EATING FOR ENHANCED PERFORMANCE

THINGS TO REMEMBER:

• Remove grain, processed dairy, and refined sugar from your diet.

• Start Monday to Friday with cheat days on the weekends. Ease into this routine.

• Food planning is useful to stay on track. Prepare meals the day before so you know exactly what and how much you are eating. Try this for the first 3 months:

  • January: Monday to Friday = Eat clean but allow 1 cheat per day (i.e. milk, cupcake, pizza, brownie, ice cream, etc.)

  • February: Monday to Friday = Eat clean but allow 1 cheat on Monday and Thursday (milk, cupcake, pizza, brownie, ice cream, etc.)

  • March: Monday to Friday = Eat clean but don't cheat until the weekend.

Note: Watch your progress. You may want to remove the cheat days sooner as this way of eating becomes more of a natural lifestyle. Use the following as a helpful guide. Fill in the blanks!

WEEKLY MEAL PLAN:

Monday: Breakfast

_____

_____

Lunch

_____

_____

Pre-Workout (Snack)

_____

_____

Post-Workout

_____

_____

Dinner

_____

_____

STEP 2: THE "WHEY" TO GO

PICTURE THIS:

You spend one hour doing your gruesome workout to get your body in amazing shape, and afterward you feed it chemicals and toxins.

After evaluating many of my friends' protein powders of choice, I noticed they used a laundry list of ingredients, half of which I did not know how to pronounce. The chemical compounds of these ingredients have become so confusing that their names are 30 letters long…

Well, if we cannot recognize the name of the food, then guess what? Most likely our bodies have no idea what it is either, and what good does that do for our bodies? As a general rule of thumb, if a food label has more than 10 ingredients written, then probably there are less-than-healthy fillers or other ingredients added you should avoid.

THE "PROTEIN POWDER" DILEMMA

First, let's first look at whether or not protein powder is even a viable product to utilize post-workout.

The question of whether protein powder is beneficial to our bodies has been thrown around by industry influencers for years—as some experts believe other sources of protein are more ideal than in a powder form. I completely understand why they are not suggesting protein powder because over 90 percent of the powders come from cows that have been treated with rBGH (Bovine Growth Hormone, which stimulates milk production), injected with steroids and antibiotics, and has been high-heat processed, which can denature many of the amino acids and other nutrients.

Protein powders that come from healthy cows with the right nutrition balance (i.e. grass-fed/organic/un-denatured sources) are challenging to find. However, when you find the right one, the benefits are huge. My recommendations for nutritious protein powders are listed at the end of this section.

On the whole, I believe that protein powder, specifically whey protein, is vital as it gives your body an abundance of amino acids to support your muscles. Amino acids are essential for the recovery process because they rebuild the muscle that breaks down during a workout. For those who are pushing their bodies in the gym and breaking down muscle, please take my advice and use a good protein powder 30-45 minutes post-workout to refuel your body with essential amino acids for muscle rebuilding.

> IF WE CANNOT RECOGNIZE THE NAME OF THE FOOD, **THEN GUESS WHAT?** MOST LIKELY OUR BODIES HAVE NO IDEA WHAT IT IS EITHER, AND WHAT GOOD DOES THAT DO FOR OUR BODIES?

Once you have found a quality protein powder that suits your needs and tastes good, look for the following three components on the nutrition label, as they are key parts of protein utilized by the body to increase muscle mass:

Leucine is one of my favorite amino acids and has been shown to increase muscle strength and improve overall performance. We talked about BCAA's in the first two steps of this book, and leucine is one of the 3 BCAA's, with the other two being isoleucine and valine.

Many studies have shown leucine and its role in the body, and all data reveals the same results: it burns fat, increases muscle, and improves performance. Researchers have noted that as few as 2.5 grams of leucine is enough to stimulate protein synthesis and get the body ready to create and build more muscle mass.

Carnitine, which is a compound made up of two amino acids, is known as the energy producer and works hand-in-hand with leucine to build muscle. Carnitine takes fat cells and pushes them into the mitochondria of cells, which is where fat is burned to create fuel.

This is important because the more fuel that is created—the faster leucine can work to build more muscle mass. All of these substances work together in a synergistic relationship to build muscle and enhance your performance as an athlete.

Cysteine and glutamine are loaded with whey proteins and are the precursors for my favorite antioxidant—glutathione. Historically, glutathione has been known as "The Mother of Antioxidants", due to how powerful it can be for the body. Even if your goal is not to put on any muscle mass or become a better athlete, you should still consider including a whey protein in your diet for this antioxidant.

Glutathione can be produced naturally in your own body, but due to many people's poor lifestyle choices in today's world, our body's natural glutathione numbers have been depleted, which has contributed to the rise in numerous chronic diseases such as heart disease, cancer, infections, Alzheimer's disease, and Parkinson's disease as mentioned in earlier chapters. Currently, over 80,000 articles exist showing the benefits of glutathione, including the use of it as a means of treatment for the diseases listed above. For these reasons, I suggest a quality whey protein source to all of my clients, regardless of their athletic goals.

So as you can see, I am very passionate about a high-quality whey protein because it has been a key element in my journey of achieving the personal goals that I started back in 2010. Through many years of research and personal trial and error, I've discovered excellent products that provide the body nutritious fuel to help people reach their goals.

As promised, here are my Top Whey Protein Powder Recommendations:

Stronger Faster Healthier (sfh.com)

Bulletproof Upgraded Whey 2.0 (bulletproofexec.com)

Pure Power Protein (mercola.com)

Mt Capra Goat Protein (mtcapra.com)

SECTION TAKEAWAY: THE "WHEY" TO GO

THINGS TO REMEMBER:

If you already take protein powder, the question you should ask yourself is:
What are the ingredients?

If you see your current protein powder contains a ton of chemicals then I would immediately toss it and begin to look at some of the brands suggested in this section.

Every product listed is clean and reliable so you don't have to do your own homework, as I have done it for you.

STEP 3: DO YOU NEED SUPPLEMENTS?

Over the years I've come to notice that every time I go to the gym, I see people putting the most ridiculous supplements into their body for either muscle gain, fat loss, or increased energy. The word supplement was originally created for products that "supplement" your body with nutrients that are hard to get from food.

However this does not mean that all supplements are made from good materials and are free from preservatives and toxins that may look good on you short-term but over the long haul will create many health issues. The problem is there are tons of so-called supplements on the market and it can be very confusing to know which ones to buy. But yes, elite athletes need supplements because it is almost impossible to get the proper amount of nutrients needed through your food in our society today.

I recommend taking supplements that are rated extremely high in the industry after doing tons of your own research. Reading this book is a great place to start your research. (Plus I have developed an in-depth list of top-rated supplements for you.)

When you are deciding on what type of supplements you want you need to consider products that are whole-food based—meaning that they are made from whole foods and are not extracted artificially, or not isolated as individual vitamins/minerals (otherwise the body has to pull nutrients from its own resources to make that isolated vitamin/ mineral usable by the body).

TOP 4 SUPPLEMENTS EVERY ATHLETE SHOULD TAKE

Since most people do not have a personal nutrition advisor readily available, I suggest you stick with my suggestions on the following pages for basic health and nutrition purposes, but be cautious when listening to the sales rep at the nutrition store. Most of the time, these national chain vitamin stores have products filled with preservatives and extra garbage that will harm your body, so I have included a list of my favorite companies for you below.

If you do not see a supplement you currently take on this list, then my advice is that you try them all because they will provide you with what you need to better your body to become an elite athlete.

For example, my favorite whole-food based supplement company is Standard Process. This is where I get my multivitamin and other supplements that are specific to me as an individual. Since I cannot assess every single person individually then it's important to choose a company such as this for your specific needs.

Here are my top recommended supplements for athletes and most-trusted supplement companies. The only reason to deviate from this list is if you receive specific instructions from your nutrition advisor.

BCAA (BRANCH CHAIN AMINO ACIDS)

If you are looking to put on muscle mass, this supplement is one of the easiest and most efficient ways to accomplish this goal. In fact, BCAA was one of my key secrets that I used to help drastically increase muscle mass in a short period of time.

BCAA's are found in beef in large quantities, but consuming excessive amounts of meat can be harmful to the body as mentioned in previous chapters. Therefore, adding natural forms of BCAA to the diet is a safe way to build muscle mass without over-consuming meat.

Amino acids are the building blocks for proteins. During a workout, the body is utilizing and breaking down muscle tissue. Then, post-workout, the body craves amino acids to repair and rebuild that muscle tissue. Therefore, it is vital to flush the body with BCAA's to strengthen your tissues—making you a stronger and overall better athlete. Every athlete that I have advised to take BCAA's has noticed a significant increase in muscle, as well as performance in the gym.

There are lots of companies that sell these products in mass production but as stated, I listed my favorite below as they are the cleanest. I usually take 4 to 12 BCAA's post-workout depending on the aggressiveness of my goal and how much weight I was lifting that day.

Food Sources of BCAA's:
Pasture Raised Chicken
Pasture Raised Eggs
Raw Almonds
Raw Brazil Nuts
Raw Pumpkin Seeds
Raw Cashews
Wild Caught Fish
Grass-Fed Whey Protein

Favorite Company: Poliquin Group

DIGESTIVE ENZYMES

Enzymes are the conductors of how the body uses vitamins, fats, carbs, etc. They are essential to a properly functioning body, especially in the gut system. The body is prepped with dozens of enzymes naturally, but because of today's food systems and high levels of stress and toxicity, our enzyme count is severely depleted. This is why those who are looking to take their health and fitness to the next level should supplement with whole-food based digestive enzymes.

Taking digestive enzymes will set you apart from other athletes and give you that winner's edge you are looking to achieve.

Food Sources of Enzymes:
Sprouted Nuts
Papaya
Avocado
Bee Pollen
Local Raw Honey
Coconut Oil
Eat a Raw Food Diet for 7 Days

Favorite Company: NOW Digestive Enzymes

OMEGA 3 FATTY ACIDS

Omega 3's are crucial to speed up muscle recovery and reduce inflammation overall in your body.

There are several studies that show how omega 3's can aid in protein synthesis, as well as increase the muscle-building pathway. The key with omega 3's is you are using a fish source and unfortunately many fish sources are made of harsh chemicals, which give you gross fishy burps and stomach discomfort.

Omega 3's are also beneficial to lower heart inflammation, which is a necessary task in our country today with all of the stress put on this vital organ from toxic food, air, and lifestyles. In fact, many doctors are looking to recommend Omega-3 Fatty Acids as an initial step before trying a pharmaceutical drug related to heart conditions.

Food Sources of Omega 3 Fatty Acids:
Wild Caught Salmon
Cod Liver
Sardines

Favorite Company: Nordic Naturals Fish Oil

VITAMIN D

No matter what your goal in life is, vitamin D should be a standard for every single person. The sun is the greatest resource for vitamin D, but if you do not live near the equator or spend a majority of your day in the sun, then adding some whole-food vitamin D to your daily regimen is an important component to staying healthy.

Many scientists and researchers believe the reason most people get sick through the winter months is because of their all-too low vitamin D levels. Adequate amounts of vitamin D have been shown to not only boost the immune system, but also prevent many heart disease and cancer-linked genes from turning on and being activated in the body.

A common misconception is that dairy products provide ample amounts of vitamin D. However this is not always the case as much of the dairy consumed by Americans has been pasteurized (heated at high temperatures) which destroys valuable nutrients including vitamin D.

After going through this entire process myself, I realized the lost vitamins and minerals from my body were synthetically added back through the dairy.

At this point, it has been my observation that vitamin D is not used by the body because it has for the most part been artificially created in a factory. If you want to use dairy as a regular source of vitamin D, then make certain that it is organic, raw, and unadulterated to ensure that all the natural components are present in the products you are consuming.

Food Sources of Vitamin D:
Wild Caught Salmon
Pasture Raised Eggs
Mushrooms

Favorite Company: Carlson Labs Vitamin D3

WHERE TO SHOP:

I recommend going to Amazon.com for any supplements and nutrition products.

SECTION TAKEAWAY: DO YOU NEED SUPPLEMENTS?

THINGS TO REMEMBER:

Deciding which supplements to use and for how long is usually a rollercoaster ride for a lot of people who don't know the difference between good supplements and bad.

Most people don't follow their supplement regimens regularly either which screws up their overall health and diet routine.

In the Notes section, jot down the supplements you feel would benefit your life the most and the quantities you need.

Remember, supplements are essential when you're not getting enough nutrients in your foods. However, sometimes you are not able to fulfill your body's requirements with food alone depending on your goals, therefore make sure you are getting what you need for mineral efficiency.

Tip: Buy a vitamin holder with the days of the week labeled so you are unlikely to miss a day. (Google "7-day pill organizer")

NOTES

CHAPTER FIVE

MOBILITY & MOVEMENT

STEP 4: SPYING ON YOUR WORKOUTS FOR MAXIMUM POTENTIAL

In April 2014, I began a 7-month commitment to completing the Ironman in Florida. It was one of the biggest challenges of my life especially since prior to my training I had completely given up on running, swimming, and biking for over a year. I was discouraged and couldn't fathom putting in the work required to compete in such a prestigious race. I knew I'd have to put all of my previous assumptions that I would never make it to finish line aside and work hard as hell to make it there.

The greatest distance I had ever completed before the Ironman was 400 meters, and that was part of my warm-up before doing CrossFit™. I knew swimming was also going to be a challenge because of my lack of motivation to swim for an hour. So when I finally decided to dive into the training (excuse the pun) I joined a swim club to help keep me accountable. Sometimes joining running and swimming groups, or gymnastics classes, helps you stay on track.

On Monday nights, we met for one hour, and a coach led group workouts at the pool. Swimming with other people was key because it pushed me to swim faster; if anyone swam too slowly, the coaches got right behind us and tapped our feet, letting us know we were about to be passed in the lane.

Here's an example of my swim workout before the Ironman:

Swim 100 meters

25 air squats

Swim 100 meters

25 air squats

Swim 100 meters

25 air squats

Swim 100 meters

25 air squats

After finishing the first 100 meters of the workout, I remember getting out of the water and being in shock watching a majority of the other swimmers do squats with less than quality form. Some people were sticking up their hips and not getting below parallel—and many people's knees were buckling. Others were doing some movements you only see in jazzercise videos. But who was I to judge, as I was pretty sore myself.

What I realized however was that even people who were in great shape (and had potentially competed in Ironman's and other competitions similar) were struggling during their workouts due to a lack of fundamental mechanics of the human body.

I wish I had a camera to video and take pictures of some of the poor posture and muscle strength that I witnessed to demonstrate how difficult these workouts could be when your body is not used to this type of training. As an elite athlete you should not only have the stamina, strength, and flexibility to make it across the finish line, but you should be able to excel in practice as well. Correct form was the problem when perfecting these movements. Now don't get me wrong, I do not fault the amazing athletes for this poor form, but rather their coaches for not recognizing or correcting their mechanics at the time of training.

Since that time at the pool, I have constantly noticed this type of poor form by hardcore athletes. Unfortunately, I see poor form in many gyms where people's biomechanics during workouts are the limiting factors for them going from mediocre to elite—and I came to the conclusion that triathletes could create massive gains for their bodies by changing their form and learning to squat effectively.

> ## AS AN ELITE ATHLETE YOU SHOULD NOT ONLY HAVE THE **STAMINA, STRENGTH, AND FLEXIBILITY** TO MAKE IT ACROSS THE FINISH LINE, BUT YOU SHOULD BE ABLE TO EXCEL IN PRACTICE AS WELL.

Triathletes don't necessarily know how to perform exercises to strengthen and lengthen muscles correctly. I believe that not only would they become better swimmers but the risk of injury during the other workouts (biking and running) would significantly decrease as well.

LEAVING YOUR EGO AT THE DOOR

Whether you are training hard for a competition, trying to lose weight, or even recovering from injury—it is important to understand that changing up your routine is essential for improvement. Remember that even the top professional athletes are required to alter their regular workouts throughout the pre- and post-season as well as per their coaches. If you don't, your body will plateau and you will not improve.

Rarely will you ever find a stubborn professional athlete not willing to grow and want to become better by finding their faults and weaknesses.

When I speak at seminars or in the office to clients, I record every talk so I can watch my performance to see how I can become better by improving my speaking and communication skills. The same can be applied to training. There is no room for egos and someone telling you constructively how to improve what you are trying to achieve is not a putdown, but rather necessary to reach your overall potential as an athlete and successful person in life. For instance, many professional athletes watch videos of their past performances to see what they need do to improve and become stronger athletes.

Take it from me, no matter what method of training you choose (lifting weights, CrossFit™, swimming, biking, running, or yoga) watching yourself perform on video is a game-changer.

In fact, LeBron James, one of the greatest basketball players of all time, famously said: "I'm coachable. If someone sees something and they think it could help me, I don't mind looking into it. Even at this stage in my career."

LeBron said this during an interview in 2015 referring to the fact that he needed to make a minor tweak to his free throws in order to improve his game. See, even elite athletes can improve and the best, most notable ones, can admit they need to make change in order to do so. LeBron expects the best from himself despite his success in the NBA— and anytime he sees an opportunity to grow he still listens and is willing to take action on the suggestion.

HOW TO SPY ON YOURSELF

My theory known as "Spying on Yourself" (or making videos to demonstrate your current movements while you workout) can be broken down into 4 tactics. I promise that utilizing these steps once a month will be a big game-changer with respect to your level of performance as you work toward going from mediocre to elite athlete. The movements can be incorporated into your workout if you have a private coach, or if you do group classes, then make some time before or after class to take this extra step. You won't regret it.

TACTIC #1 - SELECT THE TESTING WEEK

For one week, incorporate various different movements into your routine (such as squats, deadlifts, jerks, handstand pushups) to shake up the norm.

HOW TO DO THIS?

Hand your phone to someone at the gym (a training partner, a coach, a friend etc.), and have him/her record each new movement from the side and from the front while you do a few reps.

TACTIC #2 - PREP THE VIDEOS

Once you have performed all of the movements, you have to prepare the videos for analyzing. There are numerous apps out there for people who train, but two apps that I have used and highly recommend to clients are: Iron Path and Coach's Eye.

Coach's Eye sports video analysis app allows you to slow down each movement, draw lines, and screenshot positions so you can see areas you need to spend more time refining.

Iron Path bar path tracking app allows you to place a dot on the barbell and follow the path, so you know the direction of the bar. If you see the bar go too far in front of you during the snatch, then you know how much tighter you need to keep in the bar.

TACTIC #3 – HAVE VIDEO REVIEWED BY A COACH

Hopefully you have access to a skilled trainer or gym owner who knows what they're talking about who can analyze your videos and show you the weaknesses and faults of each movement. If there is not a professional at your gym who can do this task, ask someone you trust who works with elite athletes, and pay her or him a nominal fee to review the lifts. It will surely be worth your time and money.

TACTIC #4 – SET UP WEEKLY CYCLES

Now that you know which of your exercise movements need improvement, the next step is to create a weekly schedule to practice those lifts and different moves. I suggest you keep a chart or index card on you at all times with the days, movements, and areas of focus in case you have a few minutes to review. Follow this regimen for about 4 weeks. Then create another testing week going back to Tactic #1 and repeat this cycle with new movements.

Here is what a sample week would look like:

DAY	MOVEMENT	NEEDS WORK
Monday	Back squat Snatch	Knees out, ankle mobility Keep bar in
Tuesday	Day off	--
Wednesday	Deadlift	Create lever with hips, stop arching
Thursday	Clean Handstand Pushup	Scarecrow arms Stop arching back, keep core tight
Friday	Jerk	Front foot forward more

SECTION TAKEAWAY: SPYING ON YOUR WORKOUTS FOR MAXIMUM POTENTIAL

THINGS TO REMEMBER:

Now that you see the value of spying on your workouts, ask yourself:

When will you begin and which movements will you track?

The first step may be to:

List all the movements you would need to monitor and track; and then create the schedule. For example, here's how it would look on your Notes page:

MOVEMENTS TO VIDEO	RECORDED	RE-RECORDED DATE
Thruster		
Power Clean		
Kettlebell Swing		
Push-Up		
Plank Hold		

STEP 5: RECOVERY STRATEGIES FOR BETTER PERFORMANCE

Chances are you go to work every day, sit in front of a computer 6-8 hours a day, maybe skip lunch, then rush home only to eat inflammatory foods for dinner (white breads, pastas, cookies, etc.) and expect to go to the gym to work out like a professional athlete.

Wrong!

If you expect to train like someone who follows the "Eliteness Movement", then you better be caring for yourself like a professional too.

As you have already read, I have provided numerous tips and tricks on how to change your routine at home and at the gym to enable yourself to become more elite. But if you were to implement only some of my advice, I would suggest implementing these next few steps into your daily routines as soon as possible.

All of the professional athletes that I train focus heavily on recovery methods just as much as they focus on their regular training regimens. In my opinion, the reason they perform so well is not because of the particular programming developed by their coaches, or their workout routines in the gym, it's because of the things they do outside of the gym.

In other words, if your plan is to remain status quo and continue with a nominal 1 hour workout routine 3 days a week then fine. But I can guarantee that is most likely not why you picked up this book! You picked up this book to learn how to become your best athlete—your best self—and improve to be better than you were yesterday.

So here are my recommendations for elite recovery strategies:

EPSOM SALT BATHS

The magic ion = magnesium.

ATP (adenine triphosphate) is a molecule in the body that produces energy and helps you perform at extreme levels while working out.

Ensuring your body has ample amounts of ACTIVE ATP is crucial if your goal is to improve day after day. The secret is that ATP becomes active when it is blinded with magnesium. Otherwise it remains inactive and doesn't create additional energy that is essential for better muscle performance.

A study in 2006 showed that after hours of strenuous exercise, participants required approximately 10-20 percent more magnesium in order to function due to the amount of mg lost from sweating and urinary excretion. The same study showed that male athletes with a magnesium intake of fewer than 260 mg/day and female athletes with fewer than 220 mg/day could also be showing a significant magnesium deficiency.[3]

A different study showed that male athletes who supplemented with 390 mg of magnesium per day for 25 days had increased oxygen uptake, as well as total work output.[4] This is extremely important to note because so many people spend days, months, and even years, trying to becoming elite but physiologically their body will not allow them to do so due to nutritional deficiencies. Now we know why.

If creating higher levels of magnesium in the body are crucial to becoming a better athlete, then the question really is: What can I do to increase my levels of magnesium?

Epsom salt baths are one of my favorite ways to increase the absorption of magnesium into the body. I usually pour 3 cups of Epsom salts into a tub of warm water (stirring it to help dissolve quicker) and soak for 20 minutes. During a standard week, I take a minimum of two baths, and on a long or extreme workout day, I add an extra soak.

Sometimes I make the soak even more beneficial by adding drops of Arnica oil, which is a natural anti-inflammatory. Arnica comes from a flowering plant located in Europe and Siberia and has been shown to reduce the effects of high levels of inflammation, as well as pain. A 2003 study showed that marathon runners who took Arnica before and after their races experienced less soreness than the placebo group which took nothing.[5]

ACUPUNCTURE

One question I constantly ask during my workouts is "have I improved my athletic performance?" If the answer is no, then I re-evaluate and start thinking of extra ways I can change up my routine to better improve my performance ability.

In 2012, I found myself at a major plateau in my CrossFit™ training and as a result I started to get really discouraged. So I decided to implement an acupuncture component into the mix. I couldn't believe the immediate results!

Acupuncture practices date back thousands of years when ancient Chinese cultures used sharpened stones and bones for their treatments. Natural health science was completely new to me at the time, but many athletes used it as ways to recover so I thought I would give it a go.

[3] Nielsen, F.H., Lukaski, H.C. 2006. Update on the relationship between magnesium and exercise. Magnesium Research. 19(3): 180-189
[4] Endocrinol Metab Clin N Am 22:377-395 (1993)
[5] Website: http://www.ncbi.nlm.nih.gov/pubmed/14587684

Green Bay Packers quarterback Aaron Rodgers once told ESPN, "I've got to give a lot of credit to our training staff. They spent a lot of hours with me this week. They did a great job of getting me ready. This goes for my acupuncturist as well. She really helps." This public acknowledgement of acupuncture made headlines and changed the way health professionals developed their clients' recovery programs.

On January 5, 2013, Kobe Bryant posted a picture of his leg receiving acupuncture treatment, and another famous NBA player, Mickaël Piétrus, has also claimed to use acupuncture throughout his career.

Furthermore, one major study in the *Archives of Internal Medicine* (October 2012) found that acupuncture is effective for treating chronic pain. The study involved almost 18,000 patients and was a meta-analysis of 29 studies—meaning the study has high validity.

Personally, I do not have chronic pain, but I do put my body through significant amounts of stress from exercising, working a physical job, and always being on the go—which most of you can relate to. For me, acupuncture is a service I use to calm down the effects of my rapid-firing nervous system and to keep me balanced on the whole.

There are certain points on the body that help stop the firing of your sympathetic nervous system and bring it to the parasympathetic nervous system, which is the body's calming and repairing mode.

In scientific terms, the sympathetic nervous system originates in the spinal cord and its main function is to activate the physiological changes that occur during the fight-or-flight response. The parasympathetic nervous system originates in the spinal cord and medulla and works in concert with the sympathetic nervous system. Its main function is to activate the "rest and digest" response and return the body to homeostasis after the fight or flight response. So many of us stay in a state of sympathetic, which can be detrimental to our health.

The reasons why acupuncture treatments vary for each individual are because everyone's nervous systems function differently. However, if you commit to a plan and use this practice as a lifestyle choice for good health, acupuncture can be quite beneficial. I believe that if you are considering acupuncture, it is not a method that can just be done once or twice to fix a problem. Acupuncture, like other natural healthcare practices, is something that needs to be done regularly to see long-term change. Personally, it is something I will do the rest of my life.

ACUPUNCTURE IS A SERVICE I USE TO CALM DOWN THE EFFECTS OF MY RAPID-FIRING NERVOUS SYSTEM AND TO KEEP ME **BALANCED ON THE WHOLE**.

CHIROPRACTIC TREATMENT

When I think of a recovery method necessary for all athletes, chiropractic care immediately comes to mind. Everyone from professional CrossFit athlete Rich Froning Jr. to NBA stars LeBron James and Carmelo Anthony, as well as NFL quarterback Tom Brady, utilize some form of chiropractic care.

The commonality between these elite athletes (as well as the ones that I treat regularly at my office) is that when asked 'why they get adjusted' usually their answer is "to perform better" versus "to get rid of pain."

WHAT IS IT?

Chiropractic care has one goal—to gently put the spine into proper alignment so the body can communicate at 100 percent, while allowing you to perform and be your best. Now for your anatomy lesson:

The spine, which is one of the most intricate and beautiful structures of the human body, is made up of 24 moveable vertebrae. The spinal cord is stacked and protected with the spinal column; and the skull protects the brain. These two structures are the only ones in the entire body with bone completely encasing them for protection. The heart, lungs, liver, and other organs have a rib cage for protection, but no other system is completely encased and protected like the nervous system.

From the front view, the spine should be straight up and down, and from the side, there should be three smooth flowing curves. When these curves are in their proper position, the body can perform at its peak potential—and you can be at your best.

The discs that sit between each vertebrae look like jelly doughnuts and contain a cartilage round outside and fluid-filled inside, which is where the jelly sits. The longer someone exercises on a misaligned spine and creates more wear and tear, the faster these discs become destroyed and worn out.

In the case of a structural misalignment, known as a subluxation, the body becomes automatically restricted in its level of performance. Your body's range of motion becomes limited; your soft tissue becomes tighter; and your spine will not have the proper shock absorption for the discs between each vertebrae.

Therefore an athlete who puts weight over his or her head with the snatch, jerk, overhead squat, or press—or who performs any body weight movement with abnormal spinal structure—is creating a future problem. Similarly, those athletes who add weight to their arms or legs when running are risking their chances for injury because the extra amount of loading is increased.

So how do you know what your spine looks like on the inside?

The answer: Structural X-rays.

Most chiropractors that work on elite athletes take specific X-rays to track the structure of their patients' spines, so they know what to correct. As already mentioned, long-term damage to the spine creates significant wear and tear throughout the structure (your body) leading to degenerative discs and numerous symptoms, such as lower back or upper back pain, radiating pain into the arms or legs, and ultimately disc herniation. Through the proper X-rays, chiropractors can detect how worn the disc spaces are and how much wear and tear has occurred in order to put together a plan to correct.

However what cannot be confirmed on X-ray is a disc herniation or bulging discs, which is why proactively taking care of you is so important.

The athletes who come into my office do not wait until their upper or lower back hurts before getting adjusted, but rather they seek treatment proactively to prevent any damage from occurring. Remember, these strategies are what elite athletes do who sleep later than most of us, and have active jobs—not desk jobs like most of us. They also tend to eat healthier because their livelihood depends on their physical performance and they have coaches to work with daily.

I know many people may think that they should wait to see a chiropractor when in pain, but take my advice—being proactive with your body will only benefit you in the long run. It is like waiting to do mobility work or stretch only when you are hurt. And we all know the importance of stretching before and after working out.

It is a well-known fact that people who are proactive with their health and wellness are likely to be successful and "elite" in other areas of their lives as well.

INVERSION TABLES

When people ask me about items they should have at home as far as equipment, the number one suggestion is an inversion table.

Our bodies are constantly fighting the effects of gravity, and roughly 2 to 3 days a week are spent fighting that battle. The only true time we get to relax and get a break from the battle with gravity is when we lie in our beds when we sleep. Other than this rest time, the whole day of work and working out is filled with stress on the body as a result of gravity's constant pull.

Which begs the question: What is compromised when we fight the effects of gravity?

The answer: Spinal Discs

First of all, this is why I suggested earlier that every person needs to be on a regular chiropractic treatment plan—whether you're a pro athlete or not—simply because a poorly aligned spine can lead to poor health no matter who you are. And the longer a poorly aligned spine goes untreated, the more degeneration and wear and tear wreaks havoc not only on the spine but also on the discs.

These discs comprise an outer layer of cartilage and an inside layer of fluid. Think of the structure as a jelly doughnut. If I place abnormal stress on a jelly doughnut, like with my foot for example, eventually the fluid squeezes out. Similarly, this same thing happens when someone herniates a disc, bulges a disc, or slips a disc (all three terms describe the same condition.) The inside fluid seeps out of a space in the cartilage and needs to be sucked back into its place inside the disc. Therefore, thinking you can slip a disc back in place is a false statement because the disc itself is not what moves out of place, but rather, the liquid within it.

The goal is to keep that fluid as healthy as possible and contained within the discs—the healthier the disc stays overall, the taller you will be and the healthier your body will remain.

For example, you may have heard that 'we are taller in the morning'. This is a true statement because our bodies were off gravity for a few hours, which helps to open up the discs more. Interestingly, NASA has shown that astronauts are two inches taller in space, as they are not fighting the negative effects of gravity throughout the day.

Unfortunately, however, we cannot erase gravity from our existence like in outer space and we can only do so much to compensate for long sitting days, excessive workouts, and abundant travel schedules. So besides chiropractic care, which should be your first outlet to maintaining a healthy spine, I always recommend inversion tables.

Inversion tables flip the effects of gravity by literally flipping you upside-down which helps to hydrate and open up your disc spaces. This is vital to do after a workout, especially for those who do intense endurance training like running or lifting including heavy thrusting the bar overhead.

THE GOAL IS TO KEEP THAT FLUID AS HEALTHY AS POSSIBLE AND CONTAINED WITHIN THE DISCS—THE HEALTHIER THE DISC STAYS OVERALL, THE TALLER YOU WILL BE AND THE HEALTHIER YOUR BODY WILL REMAIN.

I use my inversion table every day for 5-10 minutes and have noticed overall better flexibility and I feel a lot more confident about having a healthy spine. This practice simply removes you from gravity and helps the joints recover from the stress put on our bodies throughout the day while on your feet (or siting) by opening up the discs.

MASSAGE (WITH MAGNESIUM LOTION)

By now many of you may be thinking I am off my rocker when it comes to recovery routines. Well, I hope not! Because I am speaking from experience and hoping to help you reach eliteness too!

However I will admit I am crazy about staying healthy. I am crazy about never getting hurt (or being able to recover quickly if I do) and being able to play with my kids when they grow up. I am crazy about being able to go on bike rides and runs with my wife when we go on vacation and not being limited. I am crazy about becoming such a good athlete that age will never be a factor in my progress or a nagging limitation.

And I want to help you do the same.

The final strategy that I'd like to recommend in this section is massage therapy. For the most part, massage therapy is underused and undervalued in our culture. But it has tons of benefits and as a result has been around for ages.

When we work out regularly or compromise our bodies by sitting or standing all day, our muscles can become tense. Also, when we workout we produce lactic acid, which leads to delayed onset muscle soreness. To counterbalance the negative effects of these stressors, people should get massages at least once a month (ideally twice a month) to release the lactic acid from the muscles and expedite recovery.

In fact, I am tempted to avoid using the term "massage therapy," as the term gives the perception of some form of relaxation only or a luxury therapeutic treat. Therefore, I prefer the term muscle therapy because that is exactly what it does when you go to someone who is good at administering their technique and can target specific muscles to get them to release. Further, daily stressors can create tight tendons, which are the spots where muscles and bones connect. By working on these, as well as the muscles, we can exponentially reduce the risk of injury as we age.

We also constantly hear the terms "torn muscles" "torn tendons" or "torn ligaments" which typically occur as a result of chronic tension on our bodies from hunching over a screen for long periods of time, traveling regularly, sitting for extended time frames, and so on. (The exception, however, is in an acute situation like getting in a car accident or injured during a sporting event.)

As I have reiterated throughout this book, daily stressors play a major role in the daily health of our bodies. The good news is that we have the potential to bring our health back to an elite level by taking small steps to create big change.

While of course there are different ways you can self-massage at home, the reality is that nothing replaces the magical touch of a trained "muscle therapy" professional. If you do prefer to massage at home, perhaps in between appointments, I would recommend fitness expert Jill Miller's Yoga Tune-Up balls as they provide just the right amount of pressure your muscles require to make a difference.

Keep in mind that as we increase flexibility and motion within our joints and ligaments, the more positive impact it will be for us long-term.

In the next section I specifically outline the most common areas to utilize the Yoga Tune-Up balls for ways to improve overall performance.

KEEP IN MIND THAT AS WE INCREASE FLEXIBILITY AND MOTION WITHIN OUR JOINTS AND LIGAMENTS, **THE MORE POSITIVE IMPACT IT WILL BE FOR US LONG-TERM**.

SECTION TAKEAWAY: RECOVERY STRATEGIES FOR BETTER PERFORMANCE

THINGS TO REMEMBER:

In this section, you were introduced to five different tools for better performance—as well as various healthcare providers that are integral to a healthy lifestyle.

It is important to realize that all of these elements work synergistically in order to create a healthier you and allow you to be part of the Eliteness Movement.

THE FIVE STEPS FOR OPTIMAL RECOVERY ARE:

Epsom Salt Baths

Acupuncture

Chiropractic Care

Inversion Tables

Massage Therapy

Tips:

- In the Notes pages at the end of this chapter, begin by accumulating names of companies that manufacture the products you desire and then names of providers for the services you want to acquire in your life.
- How do you do this? Well, the best way is to get referrals from friends and family, but the key is finding someone who objectively measures your progress.
- Keep in mind, some athletes may feel great without the necessary professionals helping them; but often they are in constant pain or on the verge of breaking down physically which means no more training.

Here's how I integrate healthcare providers into my week:

Every Thursday at 6:30 AM - Chiropractic Adjustment

Every other Friday at 10:00 AM - Massage Therapy

2nd Saturday of the month - Acupuncture

Nightly for 3 to 5 minutes - Inversion Table

Weekly - Epsom Salt Baths

By slowly integrating these tools into my lifestyle over the years, I have been able to make them a vital part of my weekly routine for the better.

STEP 6: THREE KEYS TO REDUCING RISK OF INJURY

When we talk about proper ways to work out without overusing injuries there are some key joints that must be addressed. When someone gets a tear in a ligament, labrum, or tendon, one of the most common causes is due to the buildup of stress on that area over time. For example, people who tear their Achilles heel tend to have poor ankle flexion and tight calf muscles. Someone who tears a rotator cuff tends to have poor shoulder mobility, tight trapezius, and tight pectoral muscles.

Many of these injuries could be avoided if the athlete were to take better care of the individual areas and keep them healthy. Most of you reading this book plan to work out regularly and intensely for the rest of your life so making sure the joints are strong and healthy will be crucial.

Below I have listed the three most common joints that I treat for injuries. In each section I have also provided specific ways that you can prevent surgeries and permanent damage.

SHOULDER JOINTS

First, evaluate yourself.

Stand up straight and relax. Assume your normal standing position and posture. Grab two long, straight items to hold in each hand. Pencils, pens, rulers, sticks will all work. Hold them in your fists and let your hands drop by your sides. Again, relax.

Your items should be pointing straight ahead, and your knuckles should be facing flat against the side of your leg. If your palms face eachother, you will notice the top of your hand is in front of you, versus to the side of you, which is incorrect. Your shoulders are probably slumping forward, and your scapular retraction most likely needs supportive work.

Next, raise both arms as if you are waving goodbye. Your hands should be about ear height, and your elbow should be bent at approximately 90 degrees. Maintaining that arm position, push your arms and elbows back by retracting your scapula.

Ideally, both arms should go back an equal distance. If one arm lags behind then you know that side of your body needs extra work.

COMMON INJURIES & HOW TO AVOID

As a healthcare practitioner, when I am asked what the most common injuries and complex joint on the body is, the shoulder is what automatically comes to mind especially for athletes. The shoulder is where the humerus bone connects into the scapula (a.k.a. the shoulder blade).

THERE ARE SIX TOTAL MOVEMENTS THE SHOULDER CAN MAKE:

Flexion

Extension

Abduction

Adduction

Internal Rotation

External Rotation

TWO KEYS TO AVOIDING SHOULDER INJURY:

Maximum mobility

Maximum stability

If you create high levels of mobility and stability, your risks of getting a shoulder injury are significantly decreased. At seminars, I strongly encourage people to always start with mobility then work on the stability.

MOBILITY TECHNIQUES

The odds are very high that the average person reading this book has a desk job enduring long bouts of sitting in front of a computer. Straining the shoulders in such a way causes their shoulders to round forward and establish poor posture. All of this physical stress creates limited levels of mobility and added pressure due to the excessive amount of cervical flexion (head beyond the shoulders).

Mobility in all ranges of motion is essential for the shoulder joint, especially during all the lifts and bodyweight movements that utilize this joint. For those wanting to be elite, spending a few more minutes on mobility is crucial, and the next section goes more into steps on how to do this.

For the shoulder there are key stretches and mobilizations that are very important before working out. Here are my top 3 go-to Mobility Warm-ups (banded motions) specifically for the shoulder:

A) BROOM SHOULDER OPENER (FRONT AND BACK)

HOW-TO:

OPTION 1:

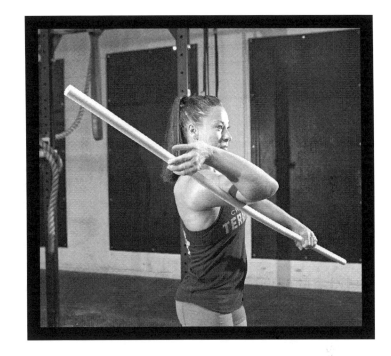

1) Place the broom or PVC pipe in front of your body so it is vertical.
2) Grip your left hand around the pipe or broom at chest level with your thumb facing towards the ceiling.
3) Bend your left elbow and externally rotate your shoulder so the broom or pipe is right behind and below the left shoulder.
4) With your right hand, grip the stick and pull it up towards the sky.
5) Hold for 10 seconds before you repeat 5 times.
6) Repeat on left side.

OR

OPTION 2:

1) Take a wide grip.
2) Perform pass throughs going forward and back.
3) Repeat this movement 10 times.

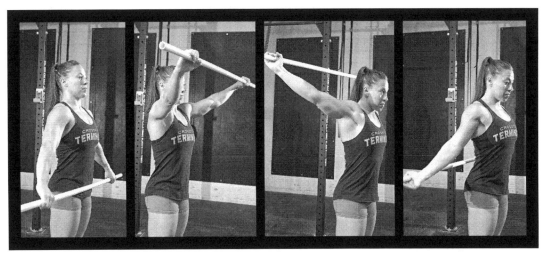

All exercise photos by Kathryn Schambach

B) YOGA TUNE-UP BALL @ SCAPULAR REGION

HOW-TO:

1) Place the Yoga Tune-Up ball behind the scapula.

2) Find a tender spot and hold it there until it reaches 75 percent maximum pain.

3) Release that spot and move to another part of the scapula area.

4) For people who would like more of a challenge, lift up your arm and bring it back down repetitively so you feel it even deeper in the scapular region.

5) Do this for roughly 2 ½ minutes per side.

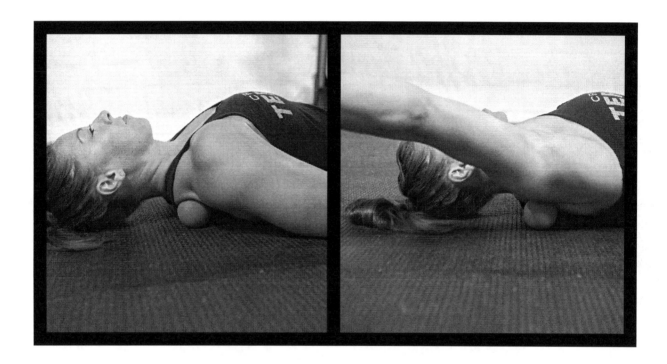

C) YOGA TUNE-UP BALL @ PEC MINOR

HOW-TO:

1) Place the Yoga Tune-Up ball right at the pec minor while you are either face down on a floor or against a wall.

2) Find the tender spot and perform circles clockwise and then counterclockwise for 90 to 120 seconds.

3) Repeat on the other side.

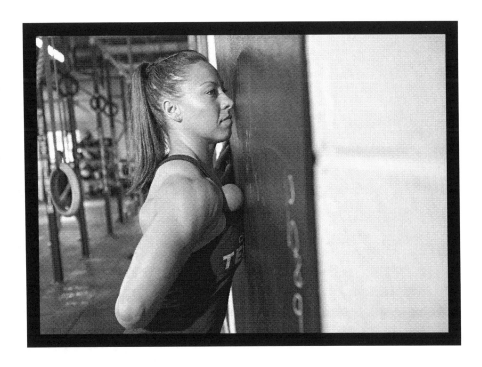

SHOULDER STABILITY

Once you have mobilized the shoulders, the next step is stabilization, or the strengthening of the muscles that support the shoulder joint. The main muscles affected are the rotator cuff muscles (supraspinatus, infraspinatus, teres minor, and subscapularis). The other muscles involved in stabilizing the shoulder joint are the teres minor and serrates anterior.

For those of you who are newbies and just made your way to a functional fitness gym either because you are tired of only running, biking, or isolated movements, or because you are interested in building elite strength—remember the transition is not directly A to Z but rather a progression of A to B to C to D etc.

The key to functional training is to work on technique and form first, and then spend time strengthening the muscles in order to progress to more advanced levels. In the CrossFit world, there is a lot of talk of "kipping", which is a gymnastics movement that uses an extreme and quick force to hoist your body over a bar. Athletes "kip" with movements like ring dips, pull-ups, toes to bar, muscle ups, handstand pushups, and so on.

The goal of kipping is to complete a workout faster. That's it! So if your goal is to be top at your gym in terms of numbers and have your name high on the board, then proceed, but hopefully you have goals beyond your times. Hopefully, you have bigger goals of creating foundational strength in order to become better at daily fundamental movements such as sitting, lifting, bending, and walking—as well as to increase your athletic ability. To me, this is the whole basis of functional training.

A major issue I see is when athletes use a "kipping" motion before they can do the movement with accuracy (or without extra movement used for momentum). For example, performing 50 kipping pull-ups before you can do five strict pull-ups is one of the worst things to do for the shoulders. Kipping is an easier way to complete the movement, but doing the strict version of the movement will perfect your technique, making it easier in the long run.

Since kipping is such a quick action, the body experiences an intense amount of immediate pressure, which tears at the muscles and joints. Continually harping of the shoulders in this way creates long-term damage that can manifest as symptoms like rotator cuff or labrum tears or otherwise sprains and strains the shoulder joint.

If you are new to a functional training program, you must go through progressions of movements before graduating to kipping. For example, for pull-ups the progression goes from supine pull-ups to banded pull-ups to strict pull-ups, and then to weighted pull-ups before finally moving to kipping pull-ups. In the case of ring dips, start with banded dips, followed by a minimum of 10 strict ring dips, and then go to kipping.

> HAVING THE ABILITY TO PERFORM MORE STRICT MOTIONS IS A **GAME-CHANGER** FOR KEEPING YOUR SHOULDER **HEALTHY AND INJURY-FREE**.

However I am OK with kipping during a competition if your muscles and joints are strong enough to handle the pressure. For training purposes, though, having the ability to perform more strict motions is a game-changer for keeping your shoulder healthy and injury-free.

The following 3 movements are excellent stabilizing exercises that build tons of strength, especially in the shoulders:

A) ABDOMINAL ROLLOUTS (5 MINUTES)

HOW-TO:

1) Set up on your knees with a barbell in front of you.

2) Grip the barbell and make sure there is enough weight to keep you up right.

3) Roll the barbell forward and backwards making sure the core is tight.

4) Do not hyperextend the lower back and make sure to stay engaged.

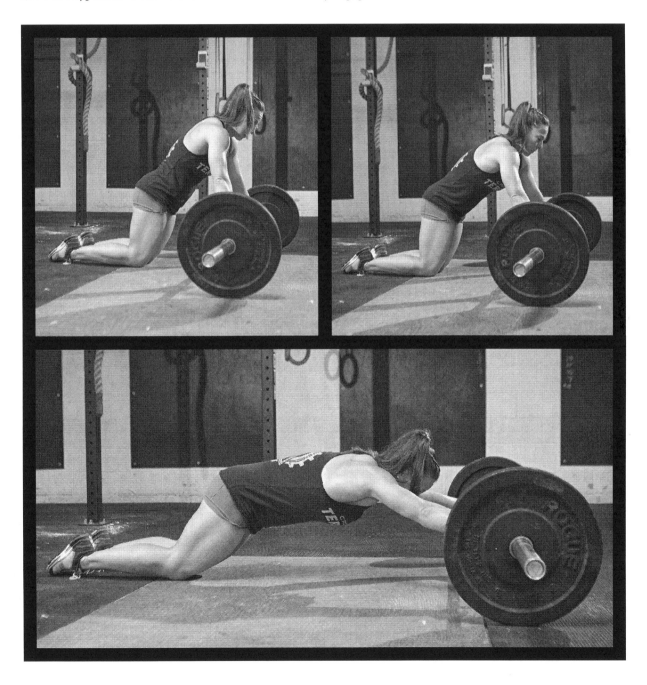

B) SCAP PUSH-UPS

HOW-TO:

1) Set up in the push up position making sure your lower back is engaged.

2) Squeeze your shoulders together so your body moves forward but arms are still straight.

3) Relax and then get back into the neutral push-up position.

4) Repeat 12 times for 3 rounds.

Scap push-ups engage the serratus muscle, which is great to keep the shoulder stabilized. In fact, the scap pushup is one of my favorite moves to do when I travel or am on the road and do not have access to a gym.

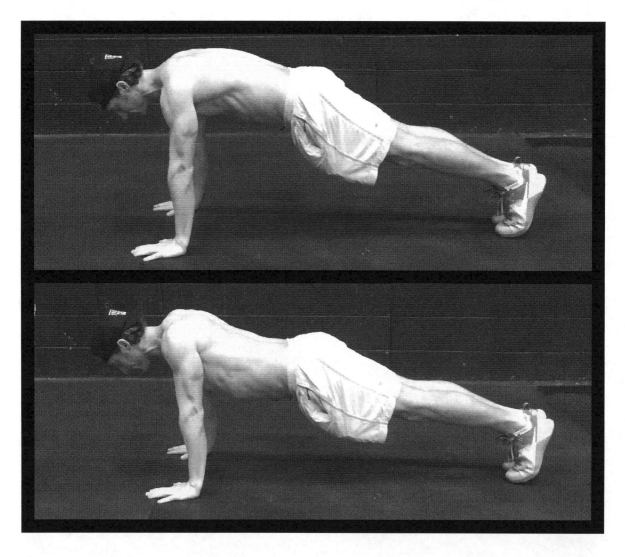

The key is simply to keep the neck, back, and legs in a straight line. Imagine them as a solid board, so that all the motion occurs at the shoulder joint.

C) WEIGHTED PULL-UPS

HOW-TO:

Grab a band or weighted belt that has a clip.

1) Place the band or weight around you and use whichever weight you feel comfortable with to start.

2) Perform strict pull-ups working toward a 1-rep max of your ultimate goal—getting to 33 percent of bodyweight for men and 20 percent of bodyweight for women.

As stated earlier, creating muscle strength in the shoulder is essential before kipping, which is especially important for those of you who enjoy pull-ups.

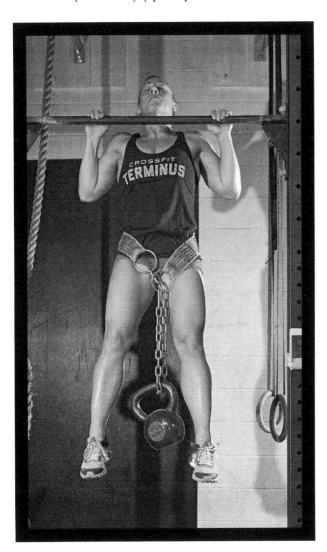

According to the OPEX Assessment Level 3 Upper Body Pulling instruction, the trainers encourage their males to shoot for a 1RM weighted pull-up at 33 percent of their bodyweight and females should shoot for a 1RM weighted pull-up at 20 percent of their bodyweight. OPEX is a global leader in coaching individuals serious about fitness and education systems for coaches in fitness.

These are definitely lofty goals for many athletes, but the journey toward reaching them is the game-changer. Keep that in mind!

HIP CAPSULE

Even though I have said the shoulder joint is the most complex, and it is where I see the most common injuries, the hip joint is the chronic joint.

What do I mean by "chronic joint"?

When people hurt their shoulders, it usually happens instantaneously, whether they tear a muscle, tendon, or ligament. Yes, for the most part this is due to a chronic lack of good biomechanics—but the injury often happens fast and immediately.

However the hip is still very different.

Think of how many hours you sit a day, especially if you have a desk job. As stated in earlier chapters, if you train like an elite athlete but sit all day, your hip mobility still decreases dramatically no matter how much training you do. It is a fact that staying in the same seated-position for extended periods of time shortens your hip flexors and weakens the gluteal muscles.

When the glutes become weak and the hip flexors shorten, this activates the lower back, which takes over the bulk of the stress. Hip mobility then shuts off and when we bend down to do something as easy as pick up an object, or use our hips in any capacity, we are unnecessarily stressing out the lower back. The even more disappointing news is that your lower back was not meant to be extremely active in these situations, as it was created to stabilize the body and be a support system for everything on top.

Unlike a tear in the shoulders from overuse that is immediate, pressure on the lower back continuously gets tighter and tighter, and you will eventually notice increased lower back pain. The more you use the lower back to compensate from 'poor hip mobility' and a misaligned upper body structure—a greater amount of stress is put on the discs between the vertebrae. An unfortunate result of that, too, is an increased risk for herniated eruptions.

Therefore once you begin to strengthen the glutes and lengthen the hip flexors, you will begin to take your mediocrity performances to an elite level. Many of the gains you will see quickly change when you take stress off the lower back will be when you perform kettle bell swings, Olympic lifts, squats etc.

The diagram to the right shows the main players in hip mobility.

From my experience working with athletes and chiropractic patients, there are three big players as far as opening up the hips. By getting the hip joint to move the way it was designed, you will immediately take a lot of stress off the lower back and improve your structural health and athletic ability.

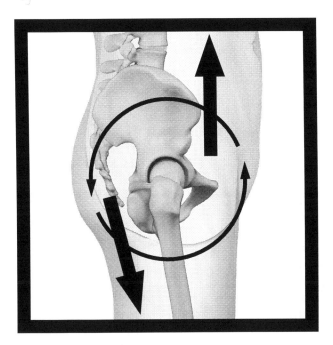 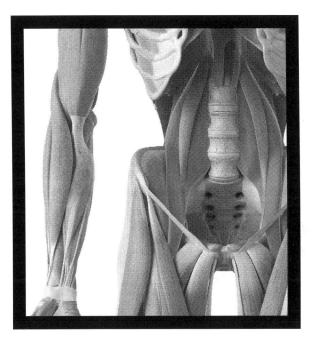

MOBILITY TECHNIQUES

The following three mobility techniques focus on these parts of the hip:

Psoas

Each of a pair of large muscles that run from the lumbar spine through the groin on either side and, with the iliacus, flex the hip. A second muscle, the psoas minor, has a similar action but is often absent.

Rectus Femurs

The rectus femoris muscle is one of the four quadriceps muscles of the human body.

Tensor Fasciae Latae

A muscle in the thigh.

A) PSOAS SMASH

Before you begin to smash the psoas—the first step is actually finding the psoas. You can see the muscle on the previous diagram, but let me help you find it first:

HOW-TO:

1) Lie on your back, and imagine a line from the bellybutton to the hip joint. Roughly 5 cm off the bellybutton is the muscle.
2) Flex hip by bringing your knee to your chest; then relax your leg back down to the floor. The psoas is a deep muscle in the stomach, and you should be able to feel it tighten and relax as you move your leg up and down.

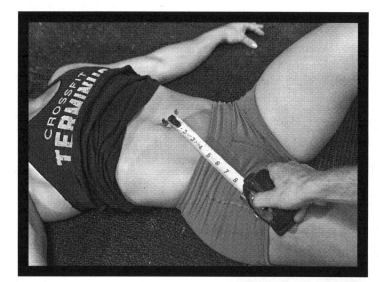

Once you find the psoas muscle, then it is time to do some work on it. This can be done in different two ways.

OPTION 1:

1) Lie on your back.
2) Place a kettlebell on the psoas muscle.
3) Take a deep breath in.
4) As you breathe out, push the kettlebell into the psoas while lifting one leg up.
5) Keep your knee bent.

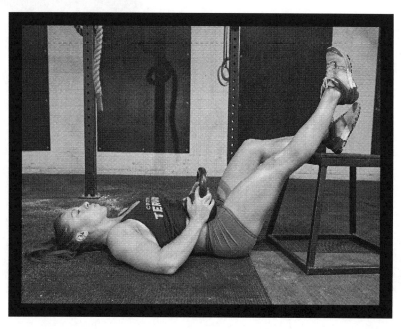

OR

OPTION 2:

1) Lie on your stomach.

2) Place a slam ball on top of your
   psoas muscle (between your body
   and the floor).

3) Take a deep breath in and then
   breath out rolling the muscle.

Note: Perform 10 to 12 repetitions of
either option so you accurately hit the
psoas and reduce its tightness.

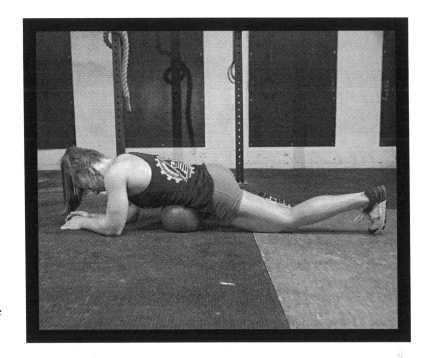

B) RECTUS FEMORIS (QUADRICEP) PULL

This move is essential for greater hip mobility regardless of the type of exercise you are doing.

HOW-TO:

1) Kneel on the ground to start.
   • LEG ONE: Bend the knee in front of you,
     so that it forms a 90 degree angle and your
     foot is flat on the ground.
   • LEG TWO: Bend the knee behind you in
     such a way that the bottom of your foot is
     facing the ceiling and your toes are against
     the wall.

2) The goal is to slide your knee as close to the
   wall as possible in order to get a deep stretch
   in the quad muscle, while also keeping your
   body upright and maintaining the other leg's
   90 degree angle.

3) Hold for 30 seconds, then switch legs.

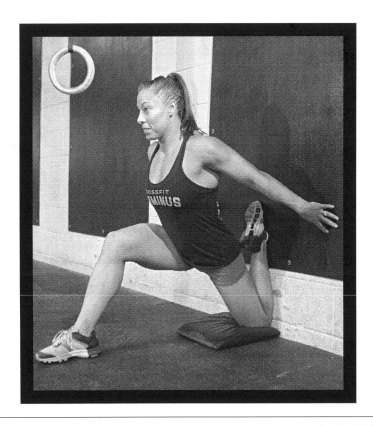

C) TENSOR FASCIAE LATAE (THIGH MUSCLE) ROLL

When people ask for ways they can release tension in their muscles, I suggest using a foam roller, which is usually followed by a negative reaction on their part. People tend to shy away from foam rolling because it can be a painful experience.

However, the problem is that most of the time they do not roll out specific muscles—and ultimately don't get to the root of the tightness. One of the reasons I wrote this book is so you know the 'why' behind what you do and how to do it.

To find and roll out the TFL, do the following:

1) Stand and put your hand flat on your hip bone with your thumb pointing down your leg (this is your TFL muscle so keep as your point of reference).
2) Lie on your stomach over a foam roller, so that the pressure of the roller is on the TFL muscle.
3) Either roll back or forth or hold the position on the TFL.
4) Hold the position until it becomes 75 percent painful and then roll off.
5) Continue this pattern 10 to 15 times in a row, then rest.

If you are looking for more ways to stretch or lengthen your hip flexors, check out author and fitness expert Kelly Starrett's best-selling book *Becoming a Supple Leopard: The Ultimate Guide to Resolving Pain, Preventing Injury, and Optimizing Athletic Performance* (Amazon).

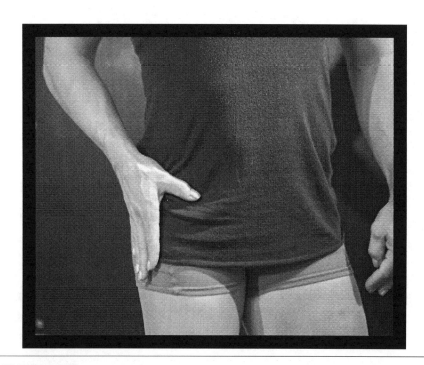

These are the major components of the hip flexors:

PSOAS MAJOR

Each of a pair of large muscles that run from the lumbar spine through the groin on either side and, with the iliacus, flex the hip. A second muscle, the psoas minor, has a similar action but is often absent.

ILIACUS

A triangular muscle that passes from the pelvis through the groin on either side and, together with the psoas, flexes the hip.

QUADRICEPS

The large muscle at the front of the thigh, which is divided into four distinct portions and acts to extend the leg.

GLUTES

Now that you have lengthened and/or released tension in the three hip muscles, it's time to strengthen the glutes. Similarly, in order to mobilize and stabilize the shoulder, the hip needs to be lengthened (stretched) and strengthened to become normal again.

The two muscles we will focus on in this section are the gluteus medius and gluteus minimus since a big problem in society today are that people are sitting way too long every day and this will eventually weaken these muscles.

What Are They?

GLUTEUS MEDIUS

One of the three gluteal muscles, it is a broad, thick, radiating muscle, situated on the outer surface of the pelvis.

GLUTEUS MINIMUS

One of the secondary muscles that can produce hip extension. This muscle is located deep and somewhat anterior to (in front of) the gluteus medius. It is a broad and triangular muscle.

Sample Glute Exercises:

A) WEIGHTED GLUTE BRIDGE

HOW-TO:

1) Lie on your back and bend your knees to 45 degrees, keeping your feet on the ground.

2) Bring your feet as close to your buttocks as possible while not compromising the lower back.

3) Grab a lighter weight i.e. 10-pound kettlebell or bumper plate to start.

4) Place the weight over the pelvis right below the hips.

5) Thrust your hips off the ground and squeeze those glutes as tightly as possible (your back should be in a straight line with your legs).

6) Hold for 1-2 seconds and repeat for 10 to 15 reps.

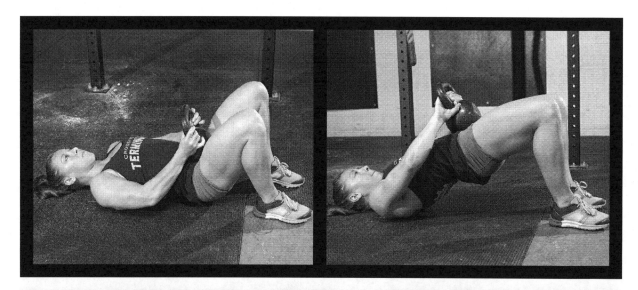

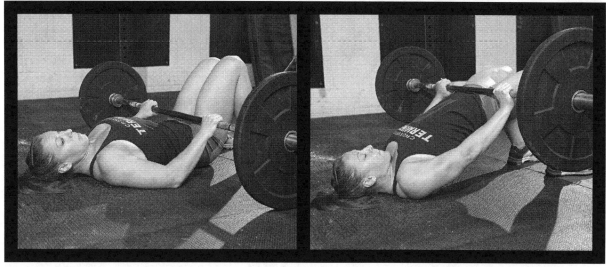

Note: As you advance in this exercise, increase the weight slightly and eventually use a bar with plates.

B) BANDED SHUFFLE

HOW-TO:

1) Use a band that gives you enough resistance. Pull it around your ankles with a tight grip on the ends of the band.

2) Get in the squatted position (not deep squat) preferably at a 90-degree angle.

3) Move your right foot to the right, following with your other left foot but keeping equal distance apart, then bring your left foot over to touch the right foot.

4) Complete 3 rounds of 10 reps each foot for this movement.

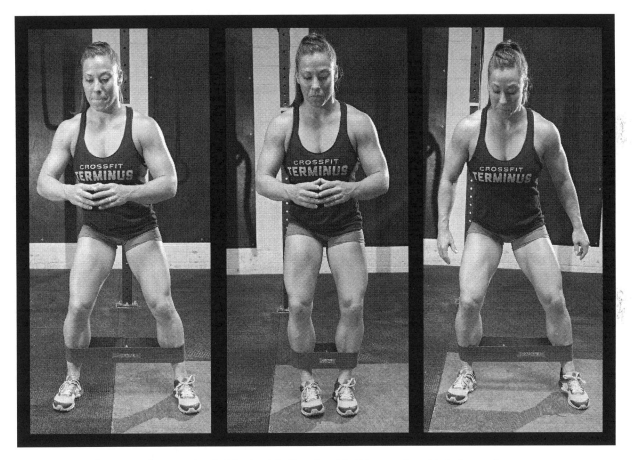

Note: As you advance in this exercise, hold a kettlebell or dumbbell in your hand to help you increase core stabilization.

C) BANDED DONKEY KICK

HOW-TO:

1) Hang a light resistant band from a rack.

2) Position yourself on all fours.

3) Extend your hip with the knee bent to 90 degrees.

4) Connect your foot to the band.

5) Drive your foot up and back toward the ceiling.

6) Hold for 1 to 2 seconds and repeat this movement 15 times.

7) Switch feet and perform two rounds.

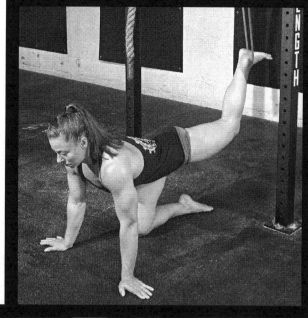

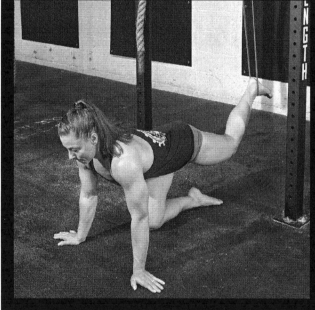

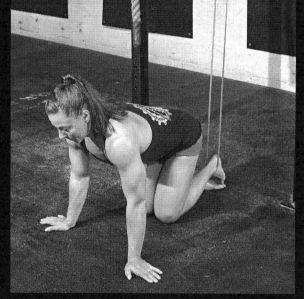

KNEE JOINTS

In the past two sections we focused on the shoulder and hip joints—and ways to strengthen and increase mobility for better performance and decreased risk of injury. Alternatively, when it comes to the knee joint, the injuries and pain that can occur are typically due to problems in other joints.

The knee is the shortstop between the hip joint and ankle joint. Conversely, knee problems tend to result from either weaknesses or immobility of one or both joints on either end. The suggested strategies for the hip (see previous section on the hip) will also be beneficial for the knee.

For example, if an athlete has a weak hip joint, the body will compensate by overusing the knee. Consequently, our bodies do whatever it takes to maintain a balanced state, both internally and externally. Unfortunately, however, that means we will more than likely experience symptoms of pain or discomfort if we are unbalanced—which is why these exercises and stretches are so important.

Some of the most common knee injuries I treat at my office are meniscus tears and ACL injuries, which are usually due to overuse and an overload of stress to the area. All of this pressure causes the knee joint, tissue, and surrounding muscles to weaken, and eventually they can tear.

Health care providers like myself—chiropractors as well as physical therapists—can provide excellent support for a patient's body, but an important component of preventing knee injuries comes down to the homework you do outside of our offices.

Here are the top ways you can decrease your risk of a knee injury or pain:

INCREASING ANKLE MOBILITY

From a young age, our parents have placed shoes on our feet as a way of protecting us from stepping on anything sharp, spiked, or harmful. Then, as we get older, many of us, especially women, increase the support in the heel of the shoe as a means for style and fashion. Doing so compromises the natural position of the foot and decreases the amount of dorsiflexion we have (dorsiflexion is a flexion of the foot when the toes are brought closer to the shin). Dorsiflexion of the foot is crucial for increased squatting, running, box jumps, and other movements we need for our ankle to be mobile.

Question: Will losing ankle dorsiflexion prevent us from getting into the squat position? Answer: No!

However, other areas of the body will have to compensate to adapt to the weakened mobility area and lack of dorsiflexion of the foot.

Can you guess which joint that is? Yes, it's the knee!

There are plenty of ways to work out with ankle immobility, but doing so ultimately masks the problem happening simultaneously in the knees. As we continue to put unbalanced pressure on our joints through improper form, especially during a workout, stress and pressure on the knee capsule dramatically increases, leading to eventual injury (and halting our ability to perform at an elite level).

Here is a test to determine your ankle dorsiflexion ability. Following is a 5-step process to maximize ankle mobility (without stressing the knee) to help you properly perform a squat or any other movement that requires dorsiflexion.

PERFORM ANKLE DORSIFLEXION TEST

HOW-TO:

1) Stand 5 inches away from a wall with one foot flat on the ground, toes facing the wall.

2) With the other foot planted flat behind you, touch that front foot knee to the wall without lifting up your heels.

3) Then, switch leg positions, and do the test on the other leg. The goal for optimal range functioning is to be able to touch each knee to the wall without lifting your heels.

4) If you are able to completely touch your knee to the wall (standing 5 inches away or more from the wall), your dorsiflexion levels are optimal, and your risk of injury is much lower than the average athlete who has lower than 5 inches of dorsiflexion.

The scale for levels of dorsiflexion is as follows:

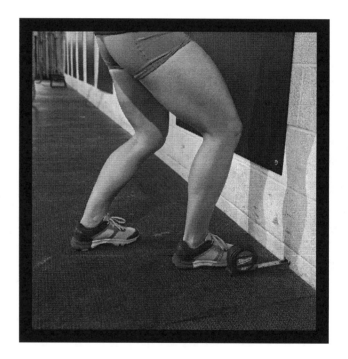

Fewer than 2 inches = Failed test

2 - 4 inches = Mediocre Levels

5+ inches = Eliteness

If you are in the failed test range or mediocre then you should continue reading the next 5 steps on how to increase your dorsiflexion levels. If you are in the "elite" level then the next few sections are still helpful.

Sample Exercises:

A) STRETCH SOLEUS

HOW-TO:

1) Place the ball of your foot against a rack (gym equipment that holds the hand-held weights).

2) Lean forward into the rack with your knee.

3) Hold the position for roughly 30 seconds.

4) Repeat 2 to 3 times on each foot.

Note: You can use a rack or anything on the ground in the gym that is raised to a 35-40 degree angle.

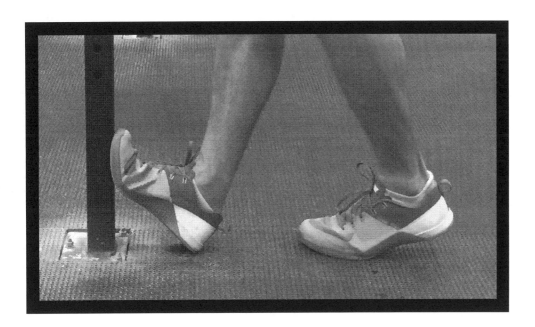

B) SQUATTED TOE LIFT

HOW-TO:

1) Place a plate on the ground and rest the ball of your foot on the plate.

2) Bend both of your knees into the squat position.

3) Repeat this movement 15 times.

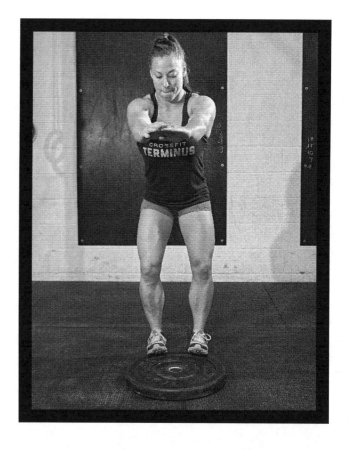

C) FOAM ROLL CALF MUSCLE

HOW-TO:

1) Lie on your back and position the foam roller at the ankle.

2) Begin to roll it under your calf holding it on tight spots for a couple of extra seconds.

3) Repeat this movement 15 times.

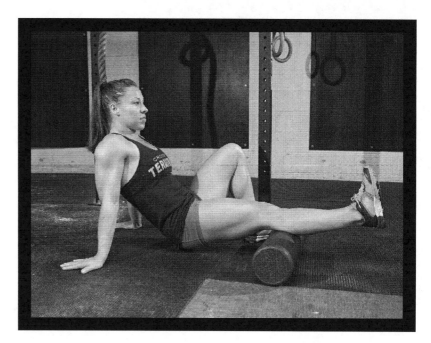

D) BANDED PULLS

HOW-TO:

1) Sit against a wall and wrap a band around the ball of your foot.

2) Push against the band and then using your arms begin to dorsiflex your foot more and more.

3) Keep doing this until you feel it has the proper amount of dorsiflexion. You may feel a slight pull or tightening but not too much.

Another Option:

1) Take a band and wrap it against the rack.

2) Place your ankle setup similar to the Dorsiflexion Test and lean forward with the knee bringing the foot more into dorsiflexion.

3) Hold this position for 5-10 seconds and repeat 5 to 7 times.

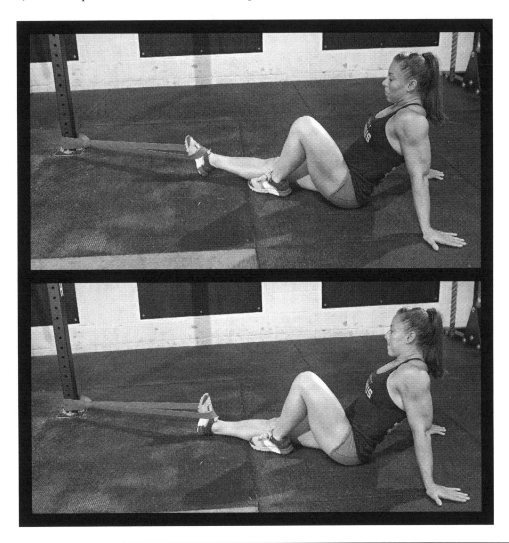

FOOT COMPLICATIONS RESULTING IN KNEE ISSUES

A) WEAK ARCHES IN THE FEET

Many people lose the arch in their feet at a young age and the amount of pronation (inward rotation) is significant. You can check your pronation levels of your feet by looking at the bottom of your shoes. If you measure the levels of wear and tear on the bottom of these shoes, you may notice the left or right side is more worn than the other. If this is the case for you, then you are over-pronating on that side, which is more than likely adding extra stress to your knees.

Personally, I have good arches on the inside arch, but the outside of my foot has lost some height over time as well as the ball of the foot. To support my feet, I have customized orthotics in my shoes, which have drastically helped my running, squats, box jumps, and other exercise movements. If you have low arches, or if you over-pronate, talk with your healthcare professional (chiropractor, physical therapist, or podiatrist) about whether orthotics can be beneficial for you.

Besides consulting a professional, there a couple of ACTION STEPS you can take to strengthen your arches and rebuild the small muscles in the foot.

1. GO TO THE BEACH

If you live on or near a beach, I suggest you take up walking or running in the sand. Walking or running in the sand barefoot is one of the top exercises for working those smaller muscles in the foot and creating strength within the arch because this particular movement utilizes more foot muscles than we typically do on a daily basis. The first time you do this, the bottom of your feet might be sore, but this soreness is good because it means those muscles have been activated.

2. SHORT FOOT EXERCISE

A simple and extremely effective exercise for the feet is called short foot exercise.

HOW-TO:

1) Place your foot flat on the ground and bring up your arch by pulling the big toe towards the heel (keeping it on the ground and making your foot shorter).
2) Then, flatten your foot again.
3) Work up to 50 repetitions on each foot and your foot strength will improve drastically, while helping your foot and knee become less stressed and more functional.

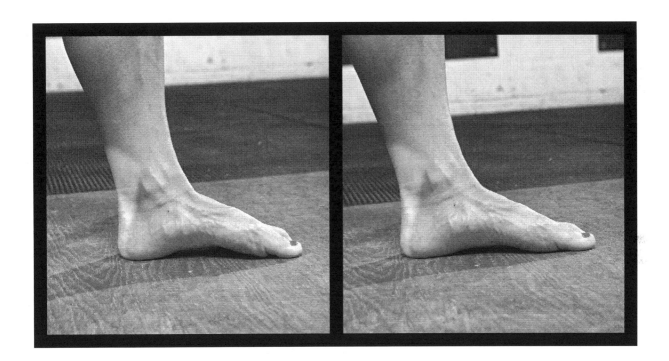

KNEE AROUND PVC PIPE

HOW-TO:

1) Put yourself in the half-kneeling position as shown.

2) Grab a PVC pipe or broom and place it right along the midline of the foot.

3) Take your knee and bring it to the outside of the stick or PVC pipe without lifting up your heels.

(Do you see how the arches rise?)

Note: Raising your arches is the goal here as it helps to build up those muscles inside the feet for better movement patterns especially with respect to running and squatting.

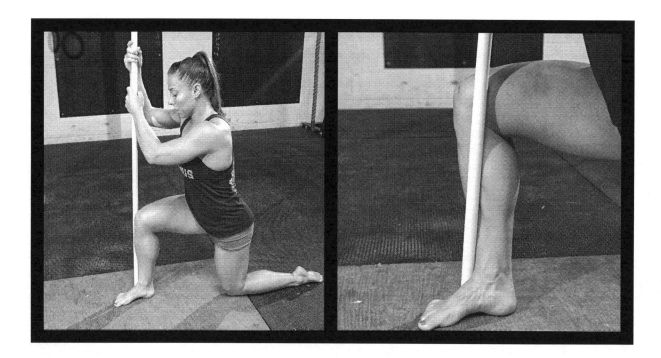

B) TIGHT HIPS

In the previous section, we reviewed the hips, focusing specifically on the most common problems that stem from sitting for long periods of time. To recap, when the hips are tight and immobile, the knee also experiences a great deal of stress because of the constant pressure, which can move the knee out of proper position.

When it comes to reducing risk of injury on the knee in relationship to the hips, the important action step is opening up the hip joint even more to make it more mobile. For those who have had previous knee issues including scope or surgeries then this will be especially important for you to add to your routine on top of the suggested hip exercises in the previous section.

BANDED HIP ROCK

HOW-TO:

1) Tie a band around the equipment rack.

2) Place the front foot at a 90-degree angle and the back foot on the ground.

3) The band will go around the back leg in the middle of the femur bone.

4) Rock back and forth with the hips to open up this joint and repeat with the other side.

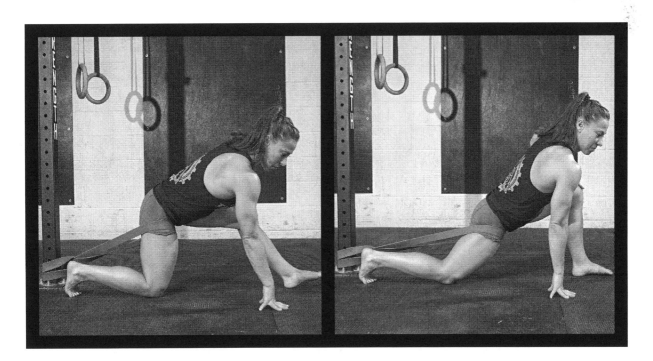

BANDED HIP OPENER

HOW-TO:

1) Start in the standing position.

2) Place a band around the outside ankle.

3) Adduct (move away) your hips from each other.

4) Turn your body 180 degrees and abduct (move toward) your hip toward the other leg.

5) Repeat this 10 times on each leg.

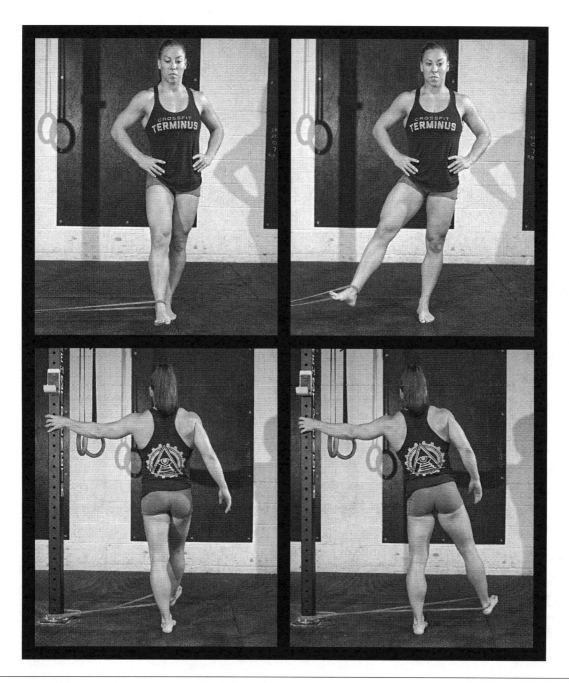

C) POOR HIP ALIGNMENT

As a chiropractor I focus a lot of my attention on structural correction. Hip alignment is such an important note to consider when dealing with preventing knee injury. Someone can do all the above exercises and stretches, but if they have uneven hips, then they are putting unwanted stress on the knee no matter what.

One of our patients, Emily Bridgers, who has competed in the CrossFit Games numerous times, came into the office because of occasional tightness in her lower back. As a collegiate gymnast, she consistently performed at high levels, and her training programs included the utilization of mobility techniques.

On her first visit to the office I discovered there was a 13mm difference between her hips from the left to the right. She never knew they were so drastically different so it was imperative that we work with her. After a short six-month program of intense chiropractic care, we re-measured her hips and her alignment had successfully decreased to only a 3mm difference. Goes to show what good chiropractic treatments can do!

SO WHAT WAS DIFFERENT?

Emily was extremely consistent with receiving care and never missed an appointment along the way. And, to this date, she has still not missed an appointment. Was she coming to the office on a weekly basis because she was in pain? No.

She was seeking out professional chiropractic care to help her perform better, make her stronger, and take her game to more elite levels. Her ultimate goal was to make it to the podium at the next CrossFit Games.
I wrote about the benefits of chiropractic care in earlier chapters and how it helps with the biomechanics and overall nerve function of an athlete. Emily's success story is a testament to what chiropractic care can provide beyond symptomatic relief.

Had Emily kept up the level at which she was competing with her hips that far off balance—who knows what the end result could have been. Not to mention her competitive career. What I do know, however, is that she has never been injured in the years she has been under my chiropractic care. Her body now works extremely well and efficiently due to proper biomechanics and nerve function.

CHECKING YOUR HIPS

The best way to tell if your hips are not aligned is to have an X-ray done and evaluated at a chiropractic office. But if you want to unofficially assess yourself at home then do the following:

Remove your shirt and take pictures of the front and back views of your body.

When looking at the back, measure the side folds (see picture below for a side fold example) of your body, and take note as to whether or not one is more prominent than the other side.

When observing the front view, look at the right and left of the bellybutton, and check to see if one side looks higher than the other.

This is definitely an unprofessional way to assess your hips. However, if you notice any indication of misalignment, then planning to have it checked immediately is crucial.

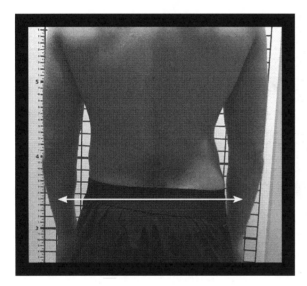
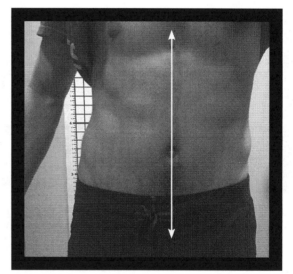

SECTION TAKEAWAY: 3 KEYS TO REDUCING RISK OF INJURY

THINGS TO REMEMBER:

This chapter may be the most difficult to grasp but possibly the most important.

Why?

Because if you talk to athletes from the 90's many of them focused mostly on their training and performance—but newer age athletes today (millennials) are focusing more on their movement patterns and mobility.

Where Should YOU Start?

> Know how each joint is broken down.
> Figure out exactly where you want to focus your efforts.
> Dedicate yourself to making change.

I suggest you jot down some of the measurements I've mentioned and use one of my favorite tools called Functional Movement Screen (FMS) to assess your shoulders and hip mobility. These tests can be found by either doing the course which I've recommended or by going online and watching an instructional video to measure the restrictions and immobility.

Note: They rank scores 1 to 3 so this way you can get your baseline for the level your body is currently. From there, the key is to track those numbers to improve performance. Use the Notes pages to track your findings. Here is an example:

> Shoulder = Right - 1; Left - 2
> Hip = Right - 2; Left - 2

NOTES

CHAPTER SIX
MINDSET

STEP 7: HOUR OF POWER

PICTURE THIS:

It's 6:00 AM and your alarm clock goes off to an Adam Levine song.

Question: What song do you sing or hum throughout the day?
Answer: Most likely it's that Adam Levine song you first heard when you woke up in the morning.

This theory proves our brains are most active first thing in the morning and the information we retain during that first hour after we wake up is the information we will probably use throughout the day.

People who strive for massive success know this principle, which is why many of them have a specific routine to start their days. Some of the most successful people on the planet who have such routines are not just successful from a financial or professional background, but they also become successful in other areas of their life: family, friendships, spirituality, social circles, community, and so on. It's how they define success beyond monetary. What does success mean to you?

Steve Reinemund, former Chairman and CEO of PepsiCo., has said he runs four miles every morning followed by prayer, reading the news, and having breakfast with his teenagers.

Steve Jobs, the late CEO of Apple Inc., once said he would look in the mirror every morning and ask himself: "If today was the last day of my life, would I want to do what I am about to do today?"

Benjamin Franklin, one of the Founding Fathers of the United States, would wake up every morning at 4:00 AM and he would shower, eat breakfast, and think about what he wanted to accomplish that day. This is what makes a successful person.

To me, individuals with a lot of money are wealthy, but they may not be very rich. There are people who are rich that do not have a lot of money to their name, but they are rich because of the joy and peace they have found in their daily lives. They are rich because every morning they wake up and live out their purposes by doing the things they love. People who are rich have a mission and vision they work towards every day and they make a difference in how they accomplish their goals.

Creating a morning routine may have nothing to do with exercising per se, but as discussed in earlier chapters, I am a firm believer in the saying: "How you do one thing in your life is how you do everything in your life." I truly believe that people who are dedicated to their health and wellness are committed elsewhere in their lives—whether that be to their families, jobs, the community or all of the above.

The reason why I am going into all of this is because in order to be a well-rounded, elite, successful athlete—you must be a well-rounded, elite, successful person in life.

HOW TO CREATE A POSITIVE MORNING ROUTINE

The first step to developing a beneficial morning routine is to make sure your two feet do not hit the floor until you have committed to your day. You might ask me: Do I wake up every single morning feeling happy, excited, and ready to dominate the day? The answer is "No way!" I am human after all, and some days I would love to stay in bed, skip work, and spend more time with my family (especially on cold, rainy days).

But, I am committed to being a successful person in all aspects of my life, so I do not get out of bed until I am happy, excited, and ready to dominate the day with positivity. Don't get me wrong, I may have to take a couple of extra minutes to remind myself of my mission for the day—which is helping as many people as I can through my chiropractic practice, spending quality time with my staff, and finding joy by being with all my patients. However, I manage to do it every day.

The bottom line is my two feet do not connect to the Earth until I have committed myself to that day. Then, once I am committed, my mind works towards my goals of exuding positive energy all day long. My morning thoughts carry me until I come home at night. And as a result, I will be in a motivated, positive state of mind for my family, which is always the most important.

Here's what my morning routine typically looks like:

TIME	ACTIVITY
6:00 AM	Wake up and DO NOT let my feet hit the ground until I am ready for the day.
6:05 AM	Jump in the shower
6:15 AM	Prepare a balanced breakfast and a cup of tea to calm the mind.
6:20 AM	Perform one of these three tasks: #1. Read a blog or two. My favorites are: SethGodin.com GaryVaynerchuk.com RobinSharma.com fourhourworkweek.com/blog pickthebrain.com/blog/ #2. Listen to a TED talk (ted.com) #3. Read a book with value! My picks are: *7 Habits of Highly Effective People* by Stephen Covey *Monk Who Sold His Ferrari* by Robin Sharma *Way of the Peaceful Warrior* by Dan Millman
6:45 AM	Review my goals for the year.
6:50 AM	Visualize exactly how I want my day to unfold both from a personal and professional standpoint—by closing my eyes and listening to soft, instrumental music. For instance, I visualize my family coming by the office to say hello. I visualize my staff excited to be at work and going above and beyond their call of duty to make my practice the highest ranked in the world. I visualize myself completing a great workout either at lunch or after work. I visualize myself with my family at the end of the day, eating a nice dinner, and relaxing.
6:55 AM	Kiss my family goodbye and head to work.

So, how about that for a well-rounded morning routine to start the day on the right foot? How different would YOUR life be if you committed this short amount of time (55 minutes total) every morning to planning your mission for the day and not letting your day's activities dictate what you're going to do or the mood you will be in?

Keep in mind of course your routine does not have to look like mine, but the key is to create a plan that is personal and meaningful to you. If it means getting up an hour earlier than the rest of your family, then that's what you should do. Losing that extra hour of sleep will not change the way you lead your life especially when your life will be more positively charged and successful in the long run.

Once you get into the habit of implementing a habitual morning routine and enjoying it, this practice will give you more abundance in your life. Believe me.

Proof is in the pudding. I treat tons of families at my office (adults and children) and they almost always ask me what my strategies are to leading a positive, successful life. I also receive numerous emails every day from people all over the world via my blog (DrAustinCohen.com) with questions about how they can lead a better life. These are the strategies I tell them. I explain to them that a solid, good routine in

A SOLID, GOOD ROUTINE IN THE MORNING IS **ESSENTIAL TO A BETTER LIFE** AND BECOMING A BETTER PERSON.

the morning is essential to a better life and becoming a better person. I also love to hear when my articles have made an impact on other peoples' lives too.

BE MINDFUL AS WELL AS PHYSICAL

It's important to note that the mind plays a key role in our health. Training is not always physical. In my experience people who constantly stay in a negative place and lack confidence in their abilities tend to plateau more often and increase their risk of injury due to high levels of stress. This book was not only intended to help you become better at the gym through eating and mobility, but the lessons I've presented are meant to serve as another tool to build titanium strength as a person, both physically and mentally.

Imagine being at peace every day on a constant uphill, never plateauing, and always knowing your life is in a state of progression. As discussed in earlier chapters about the seesaw, I encourage you to ask yourself: "Is your morning routine making your life better or making your life more of a challenge?" If your answer is the latter, it's time to change up your morning routine, which will ultimately change your perspective on life.

SECTION TAKEAWAY: HOUR OF POWER

THINGS TO REMEMBER:

This important section needs to be followed consistently in order for it to be an integral part of the process. But once it is, you will notice a big difference immediately.

How Can This Be Done?

You need to decide what an ideal morning routine looks like for you—one that will be sustainable for your life. You have read my routine in this chapter and how much I can accomplish in one hour in the morning. The trick for you will be to find what works best for you.

Your routine can either be 15 minutes, 30 minutes, or 60 minutes, but essentially you are taking that short time to focus on YOU and YOUR goals.

Your morning routine is key to living the eliteness lifestyle!

STEP 8: SEEING IS REALLY BELIEVING

Of course I can share several tangibles with you about how to become a great athlete, but the strategies that separate the elite from average are the intangibles. The elite are doing things the average gym-goer is not willing to do, such as constantly forming new habits; they work with excellence in all areas of their lives, as the status quo is not good enough for them. They keep striving and succeeding.

One major component behind these elite strategies that I tell my clients is the importance of Visualization.

At the CrossFit Games in 2014, I had the pleasure of speaking to elite athlete Dimitry Klokov and I asked him: "What do you think of when you close your eyes for those five seconds before you lift?" And he said: "I visualize myself at the end of the lift and what position I want my body to finish in."

He also added: "If I only think about the initial pull, then that will be good. But if I take myself through the lift and see myself completing it perfectly, then it will be a good lift." Dmitry Klokov won a gold medal in weightlifting at the 2005 World Championships and the silver in Beijing at the 2008 Olympics.

What Klokov may not have realized at the time is that there is actual scientific evidence that proves his visualizing techniques work.

In 2004, a study[6] was conducted on brain patterns of weightlifters that lifted hundreds of pounds and others who only imagined lifting the same amount of weight. The study tracked brain signals during visualization exercises to see if this practice could improve performance, specifically with weightlifting. The results were astonishing. The team from Cleveland Clinic found a 30 percent muscle increase in the group that went to the gym and a 13.5 percent increase in the group that only visualized their results. To reiterate, the people who did absolutely no physical activity still managed to achieve physical gains without even touching a weight.

Imagine what the results would be for the athletes who do work out rigorously and who ALSO use visualization techniques. Wow! If your goal is to be YOUR best version of yourself, then my advice is to do what the successful athletes do—visualize what you want to achieve first.

Dr. Biasiotto at the University of Chicago conducted one of my favorite studies where he split people into three groups and recorded the number of free throws each group made. He then instructed the first group to practice free throws every day for one hour. The second test group was told to only visualize making free throws, and the third group did nothing to increase the number of free throws they could throw.

[6] Ranganathan VK, Siemionow V, Liu JZ, Sahgal V, Yue GH. (2004). "From mental power to muscle power-gaining strength by using the mind." Neuropsychologia, 42, 944-956

After 30 days, he tested the groups again and guess what?

The first group improved their shots by 24 percent.
The second group improved by 23 percent without touching a basketball.
The third group did not improve at all, which was expected.

Similar to the weightlifters, the basketball players who visualized their success and the free throw going into the hoop improved their physical performance by 23 percent. This was a 1 percent difference compared to the people who actually put a ball in their hands and shot free throws on a regular basis.

So it's not surprising that one of the greatest NBA coaches of all time, Phil Jackson, constantly had his players visualize their success before games. As a team, they practiced specific mental exercises regularly so they could see themselves winning and achieving greatness. In Coach Jackson's famous book, *Sacred Hoops*, he shared that during halftime at games, he would often take his team through visualization exercises, (which he called the "Safe Spot") with the purpose of calming down the players and preparing them mentally as well as physically for the second half.

The greatest part about this intangible is that it can be used beyond athletics as it has the potential to create positive change in your personal and professional lives.

PROVEN VISUALIZATION TECHNIQUES

As mentioned in pervious sections, in the mornings I take myself through a 3-minute visualization exercise where I start by closing my eyes. I envision the coming day's events and how I would feel happy knowing that I accomplished everything I wanted that day. It would go something like this:

"Today I am going to show up at the office and hear great music playing. My great staff will be extremely excited to work today and want to transform people's lives. The first patients come early because of their excitement to get a chiropractic adjustment, and they bring a friend with them to get checked, as well. The flow of the office is flawless, the energy is high, and the phones are constantly ringing. When the patients come into the office, they share how much chiropractic care has made an impact on their lives and how happy they are with their changes in health and mobility. I go to lunch with a friend and we catch up on the great things going on in both of our lives. I start my second shift at work, and the energy is still pumped up from the morning. We carry this momentum throughout the rest of the day and treat many clients. When I get home, my wife and daughter are waiting for me. My wife is cooking a great, healthy meal as she always does, and I am fortunate to spend quality time with my family for the rest of the night. Then I will go to bed feeling satisfied with what I have accomplished during the day and look forward to the next."

Many athletes use or have used visualization techniques as part of their routines to become successful. As stated earlier, people who are willing to try something outside of the box to achieve results to become better than status quo, will always succeed far greater than those who do not want to leave the box.

Here are some elite athletes who use these techniques:

Michael Jordan used visualization to become arguably the greatest basketball player in history. He would use visualization during practices and envision the ball going in from the free throw line as well as making other difficult shots. He would do this without actually shooting the ball but by seeing it. To see is to believe.

Pro golfer **Jack Nicklaus** has described how visualization during tournaments has helped him win a lot in his career. Jack would close his eyes before swinging the club and visualize the shots going down the fairway, getting close to the pin, and ultimately going in the pin. He has won a record 18 professional majors and is considered the best golfer in history.

Tiger Woods was taught how to visualize by his father when he played golf as a child. He visualizes exactly where he wants the golf ball to go—and that's where 9 times out of 10 is goes. Tiger Woods used visualization to become arguably one of the best golfers in the world.

Arnold Schwarzenegger, five-time Mr. Universe and four-time Mr. Olympia, admits not only using visualization for his athletic success, but also credits it for his successful movie career. "When I was very young I visualized myself being and having what it was I wanted. Mentally I never had any doubts about it."

America's sweetheart **Mary Lou Retton** is one of the greatest female gymnasts of all time. She was the first American athlete to win the all-around gold medal in the Olympic Games in Los Angeles. *Time Magazine* reported in an Olympics cover story: "On the night before the finals in women's gymnastics, famous athlete, Mary Lou Retton, then age 16, lay in bed at the Olympic Village mentally rehearsing her performance ritual."

Even famous actors and people in the public eye are known to utilize visualization.

When actor and producer **Jim Carrey** was just starting out in Hollywood, he was completely broke and out of work. He decided to write himself a check for ten million dollars and dated it for Thanksgiving 1995. On the bottom of the

> # PEOPLE WHO ARE WILLING TO TRY SOMETHING **OUTSIDE OF THE BOX** TO ACHIEVE RESULTS TO BECOME BETTER THAN STATUS QUO, **WILL ALWAYS SUCCEED FAR GREATER** THAN THOSE WHO DO NOT WANT TO LEAVE THE BOX.

check he wrote: "For services rendered". He carried the check around in his wallet and looked at it every day. And low and behold, six months before Thanksgiving of 1995, he was paid ten million dollars for his work on a film. It wasn't long after that he became one of the highest paid actors in Hollywood—earning over twenty million per movie.

SECTION TAKEAWAY: SEEING IS REALLY BELIEVING

THINGS TO REMEMBER:

Sometimes when people read this section of the book, the feedback I hear is that it seems kind of hokey pokey—but the more I explain to my athletes about its relevance, the more they understand how it works to their advantage.

To reiterate visualization:

Pro MLB player Gordon Beckham's sports psychologist said it works for Beckham when he visualizes his pitches and sees himself hitting the ball.

This is very common for baseball players and other pro athletes especially when they're in a slump and this simple act can help them become a better hitter.

TO-DO:

In the Notes pages, write out three visualizations that you hope come to fruition.

Here are a few examples of what you could write:

Visualize yourself getting stronger lifts in the gym.
Visualize yourself at a certain running pace if training for a race.
Visualize yourself closing deals if you work in sales.
Visualize your kids loving you and thinking you're the best parent in the world if you have kids.

The list could go on and on, but you get the idea. Think of areas in your life that need work and begin to see those flaws turn to victories.

STEP 9: GETTING MAXIMUM SLEEP

One of the most underrated health strategies that most people take for granted (although really should be making their number one priority) is sleep. Adequate sleep can propel your athletic success to even higher levels.

The truth however is that we live in an over-worked, over-stimulated, over-technological, extremely sleep-deprived society. According to a 2014 CDC Report there are 50 to 70 million sleep-deprived Americans. This is an extremely sad statistic in my opinion, because sleep is the defining factor for resetting and repairing our bodies for the next day.

Unfortunately during my career, I have heard numerous people make ignorant comments such as, "You can sleep when you're dead." In other words, most of these people probably work extremely late hours in their jobs and rise early in the morning because their philosophy is to maximize time on this Earth. Sleep obviously seems to be irrelevant to them. Now don't get me wrong, I understand why someone would try to maximize their time here on Earth, but the honest truth is that we need to reconsider the value we place on sleep in order to do so.

Numerous studies have shown that people who get sufficient amounts of sleep (minimum 8 hours) are more effective at their regular activities and are usually more productive. Research also says that people who do not get proper sleep are more prone to chronic diseases. Therefore, if you want to wait to sleep when you are dead, then you may actually be expediting that process of leaving this fine Earth much sooner than you think. Think about that.

It is my guess that most of you picked up this book because you want to become a better athlete, and your goal is to be stronger (athletically, physically, and emotionally) than you were yesterday. One thing I can assure all of you is the best of the best athletes all value their sleep and make sure to get the minimum of 8 hours each night. Some athletes even manage to get more than 10 hours of sleep per night. They make sleep a priority in their routine.

Below are six elite athletes and the number of hours they sleep per night.

ATHLETE	HOURS OF SLEEP[7]
Roger Federer	11 to 12
LeBron James	12
Larry Fitzgerald	10 to 11
Usain Bolt	8 to 10
Andy Murray	12

[7] Sleep Source: ESPN http://espn.go.com/blog/playbook/tech/post/_/id/797/sleep-tracking-brings-new-info-to-athletes

In my experience, most people have a million excuses as to why they cannot get a minimum of eight hours of sleep every night. Some are them are:

> "I have kids…"
>
> "I work too late…"
>
> "My spouse keeps me up…"
>
> "I have a hard time falling asleep…"
>
> "I have too much to do…"

OK I get it! We're all busy and we all have a million things on our minds. But come on! I'm a parent and I have a wife, busy social life, and my own company—and I still find the time to get 8 hours of sleep each night. Remember, we must prioritize sleep and make sure it's in our daily routines (literally on our list!) because sleep is so vital to the proper functioning of our bodies.

A typical night for me includes going to bed between 9:00-10:00 PM and then waking up the next morning at 6:00 AM to do my morning ritual (see previous chapter). Do I always get a full 8 hours? Of course not!

Hey, I have a life and sometimes I'm required to stay up late. Just as in your life, various personal and professional circumstances will prevent a normal bedtime routine at times, such as going out with friends, a late work event, concert with my wife, etc.

However for me, I try to keep to a regular sleep schedule at least 5 nights a week, and if somehow I miss a night, then I will make sure to get an extra hour of sleep the following night. (Later in this chapter, I offer my top strategies to get better sleep at night.)

WHAT THE PROS SAY ABOUT GETTING SOME SHUT EYE

When I ask some of my clients (elite CrossFit Games athletes, NBA, MLB, and NFL players) what some of their success secrets are, they almost always say that sleep is near the top.

Mark Rosekind, PhD, President of Alertness Solutions and a former NASA scientist, says this about lack of sleep: "We know that sleep loss is going to create significant detriments in performance. There are lab studies that show if you're an eight-hour sleeper and you get six hours of sleep, that two-hour difference can impact your performance so that it equates to how you would perform if you had a 0.05 blood-alcohol level."

Imagine then what this means for the people who say, "I will sleep when I am dead." According to Dr. Rosekind, they are in fact living their lives and performing similarly to someone who has a .05 blood alcohol level. If these people become more serious about their sleep—one of the key factors to better performance—then they could be living even more fully each day.

As far as athletics are concerned, one study tracked the Stanford University basketball team for several months, and during that time players added an average of almost two hours of sleep a night. The miraculous results showed that the players increased their speed by 5 percent; their free throws were 9 percent more accurate; they had faster reflexes; and they felt happier overall.

These results are huge! In other words, they were not practicing any more during the study than they were before the study. They advanced only by adding two more hours of sleep each night.

HOW EXCITING DOES THAT SOUND TO YOU?

Furthermore, Harvard Medical School reported that "the body's major restorative functions" such as muscle growth, tissue repair, protein synthesis, and growth hormone release occur mostly, or in some cases only, during sleep."

> SO THE KEY FOR YOU IS GOING TO BE **CREATING NEW PATTERNS AND PROGRAMMING YOUR BODY AND MIND** TO SHUT DOWN SO YOU CAN FALL ASLEEP EARLIER AND EASIER.

The best part about this news (compared to the previous steps given in earlier chapters on how to become a better athlete) is that I am not asking you to do anything more except for shut your eyes and close down your mind for two more hours a night. Your sleep should be a high priority along with your nutrition and training regimen.

Now I get that some of you have difficulty falling asleep once your head hits the pillow and even though you want to fall asleep perhaps you can't. So the key for you is going to be creating new patterns and programming your body and mind to shut down so you can fall asleep earlier and easier.

Will this process take time?
YES!

Will it take work?
YES!

Consistency is imperative. But rest assured (excuse the pun) if you implement these strategies, the easier it will be for you to fall asleep.

TIPS ON HOW TO GET BETTER QUALITY SLEEP AT NIGHT

1. BLACK OUT YOUR ROOM

Turn off all lights in your room, so NO light is entering your eyes. Make sure your alarm clock, cable boxes, house alarm, and other devices are covered in black tape, so you do not see any light. When our eyes detect light, they block the release of melatonin, which is the hormone that puts us to sleep.

This particular reaction of the body (to wake up when exposed to the light) is actually an incredible function of the body because it enables us to stay awake during the day. But in today's technology-driven world, small LED lights are everywhere, and they are wreaking havoc on our quality and quantity of sleep. A trick I use is putting black electrical tape over the small lights in my room, which blocks the light from shining in my eyes when I am heading to bed. I have noticed a dramatic improvement in the quality of my sleep since implementing blackouts.

Besides blacking out your room, make sure to put your phone away before you go to bed because when your brain is engaged with a screen, the light blocks your body's ability to fall asleep. A 2008 study funded by mobile companies found that people exposed to a cell phone before bed took longer to fall asleep and spent less time in deep sleep patterns.

The brain needs to believe it is dark outside to start releasing melatonin, so turning off technology will get you into REM sleep much faster.

2. PUT A PILLOW BETWEEN YOUR LEGS

For those of you looking to get the best sleep ever with proper biomechanics, then sleeping with a firm pillow between your legs helps to stabilize the pelvis. When many of us side-sleepers sleep without a pillow between our legs, the hips rotate towards the mattress, which jeopardizes the structure of the spine and puts it in compromising positions.

Take it from me—a professional chiropractor with years of experience seeing patients with backs that need adjustments—we should all pay more attention to the way we sleep because 33 percent of our lives are spent resting. So grab a firm memory foam pillow, and put it between your legs to keep your body stable without putting your spine and pelvis at risk for improper rotation.

SECTION TAKEAWAY: GETTING MAXIMUM SLEEP

THINGS TO REMEMBER:

As stated in this section, a 1/3 of your day is spent sleeping.

Here's something you can do to ensure you get enough sleep:

Write out what you think needs to happen in order for you to get the best night's sleep.

Do you need to black out your room?

Do you need to take magnesium?

Do you need a new pillow?

Use the Notes pages at the end of this chapter to jot down your thoughts.

Rip your notes out of this book and keep them next to your bed so you can track the quantity and quality of sleep throughout the night.

NOTES

CHAPTER SEVEN

ATHLETE CASE STUDIES

When discussing how to push your body both physically and mentally to it's capacity in order to achieve greatness in everything you do—it is important to highlight some real-life people who have joined the Eliteness Movement already and have succeeded in pushing their boundaries.

Below are a few examples of athletes that I have worked with one-on-one at my chiropractic practice and who have reached "elite" status through this program. I help many of my professional athletes with the nutrition, mobility, and mental aspect of becoming elite, and therefore they are able to stay in that one percent of their absolute ability. The strategies that keep them on top are the same strategies that I am sharing with you in this book.

ATHLETE #1
GORDON BECKHAM, MLB PLAYER

Gordon comes to me for chiropractic services and takes advantage of many of the suggestions outlined in this book. In fact, I was told that his sports psychologist also reiterated to him what I have suggested about visualization with respect to hitting the ball and he has noticed tremendous gains from the mental aspect of eliteness.

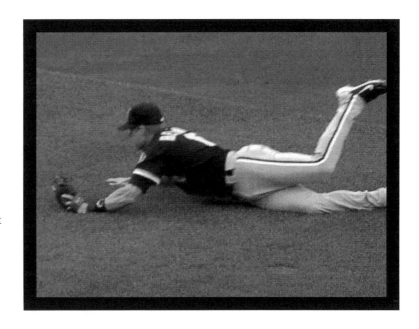

Gordon has been athletic all his life—such that of any athlete who makes it to the big leagues. He played baseball and football in high school, and was named Free Safety his Junior year and all-state QB his senior year. He signed a scholarship to play baseball at University of Georgia and played three years at UGA before he was selected in the first round (8th pick overall) by the Chicago White Sox. Gordon played seven seasons in the MLB—almost all of his career with White Sox. He was then traded to the Angels in 2014 and went to the playoffs.

Although Gordon doesn't take any sports supplements regularly, he does make sure to drink a milkshake with protein after each workout in order to refuel his muscles. As far as how he prepares for his intense training days and games, he reads his Bible every morning (part of his morning ritual; see previous chapters on how to implement a morning routine into your life).

Gordon uses contrast bath therapy during the season when his legs start to feel "heavy"—this technique is also known as "hot/cold immersion therapy", which is a form of treatment where a limb or the entire body is immersed in ice water followed by the immediate immersion of the limb or body in warm water. This procedure is repeated several times, alternating hot and cold.

Gordon also stretches before and after every workout because he seems to get very tight in his hamstrings and lower back. "I also will do wall series with a med-ball to keep the rotation that my sport requires. So stretching for me is paramount."

As for visualization exercises, he likes to envision his pitches as well as how he is going to hit the ball. "I try to visualize everything, such as walking to the plate, taking my practice swing, seeing the pitch, and taking the right swing," he explains. "I like to take it even further and visualize the ball fly into the field when I'm at bat. The same goes for when I'm playing defense, which is my forte. I like to visualize the ground ball before it is hit and think about the steps I would take to the ball and how I will use my hands to catch the ball and get rid of it. If you don't visualize what you are going to do then it almost always comes as a shock when it actually happens. If you prepare yourself mentally then you will be prepared for whatever comes your way."

ATHLETE #2
STACIE TOVAR, CROSSFIT ATHLETE

Stacie Tovar grew up in a small agricultural community of 700 people in North East, Nebraska. As the second oldest, she was raised helping out on her family's farm alongside her two sisters, and brother. "We were always an active family growing up so outside of the normal sibling rivalry and farm chores, I stayed busy playing sports," she says. "I was involved in gymnastics, volleyball, basketball, softball, and track for the majority of my adolescent years. I remember as a kid, I was always inherently athletic so I often beat the boys in my class in most activities."

In high school Stacie went on to become a standout athlete in volleyball and track, and received several scholarship offers to run track in college, but ultimately grew to love volleyball the most. She eventually accepted a scholarship to play collegiate volleyball for the University of Nebraska at Omaha. In 2008, almost two years after graduating from college and leaving competitive sports behind, she discovered CrossFit. And the rest is history!

Stacie says she takes a fish oil supplement, in addition to a protein supplement, and a post-workout recovery protein supplement. "Since I started taking fish oil about four years ago, I've noticed a significant improvement in my joint health. Consuming a daily protein supplement has allowed me to maximize my strength gains in the form of muscle mass. The post-workout recovery supplement allows me to recover faster after my workouts," she explains.

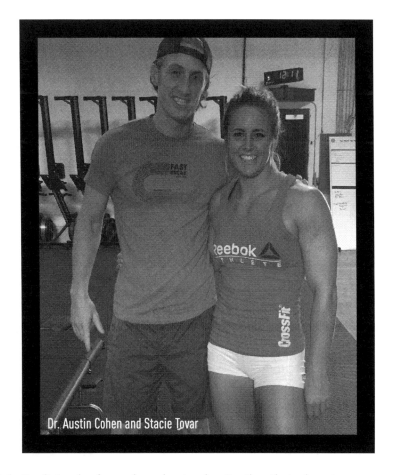
Dr. Austin Cohen and Stacie Tovar

"Regarding the post-workout supplement, I take it religiously after each workout and notice the effects almost immediately after consumption. My muscles feel like they are being replenished and refueled within minutes."

Her choice brand of supplements is Progenex. "I have literally tried a million other protein and supplement brands over the years and nothing compares to the quality of Progenex in my professional opinion."

When it comes to her nutrition regimen, Stacie is a huge advocate for healthy diets and not putting crap in her body. "You truly are what you eat. If you want to perform well, maximize your training, and look good as a byproduct then you have to pay attention to what you consume on a daily basis. Healthy eating is just a way of life for me."

Stacie tells people all the time that there really is no "one size fits all" when it comes to diet. She says for the most part she follows the Paleo diet or whole natural foods as much as she can. "I don't count calories and I don't weigh my food. I eat when I'm hungry and stop eating when I'm not hungry anymore. As an extremely active athlete, I eat to perform. I can't perform at my best if I make poor food choices or don't eat enough."

Stacie says she reads a lot of books and has grown fond of renowned sports psychologist, Dr. Jack Starks. He has a FOCUS technique that she uses often, both on and off the competition floor, as well as some great relaxation tips. Over the years, Stacie has learned the importance of harnessing her energy leading up to competitions. "Anxiety and nerves will eat you alive if you let them, so it's important to stay cool, calm, and confident as much as much as you possibly can."

As part of her regular routine, Stacie makes sure to get at least 9 to 10 hours of sleep each night. "I get adjusted by a chiropractor weekly, and see a massage therapist weekly. Outside of these requirements, I also schedule additional maintenance, which includes laser treatment, graston, acupuncture, dry needling, e-stim, or ultrasound as needed. But I notice a huge difference in my training and recovery when I don't get good quality sleep."

Stacie definitely knows what it takes to become an elite athlete, but she doesn't dismiss the fact that it takes a lot of hard work and preparation. "You have to make sacrifices. Your mental game needs to be in check. Physically, you have to be prepared to push yourself and get uncomfortable. You have to make sure to get plenty of sleep at night. Your nutrition has to be dialed in. You have to be disciplined and willing to make the extra efforts necessary to eat clean. You have to have a good support system. Surround yourself with a team of people who will either support you 100 percent or join you on your fitness journey—because you will need a positive and supportive atmosphere to get where you're going.

ATHLETE #3
DOLVETT QUINCE, CELEBRITY TRAINER

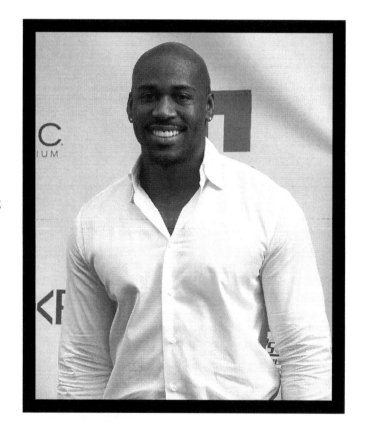

Before he became a household name, popular fitness expert Dolvett Quince endured a difficult childhood. Along with his siblings, he grew up in the uncertain foster care system and was later adopted by a Jamaican couple. However, his trying upbringing did not deter him from following his dreams in the fitness industry.

Through lots of hard work and perseverance, Dolvett followed his passion for leading a healthy lifestyle. Today he is a recognized celebrity trainer and Atlanta's "go to" master trainer. Some of his experience includes:

- Fitness trainer on NBC's "The Biggest Loser"
- Appearances on NBC's "Stars Earn Stripes"
- Has worked with many A-list celebrities including Justin Bieber
  (Dolvett accompanied the singer on his tour and created his nutrition regimen)
- Published his first book entitled *The 3-1-2-1 Diet* (2013), which outlines a healthy lifestyle model
  with complimentary exercises

NUTRITION AND SUPPLEMENT REGIMEN

Dolvett follows a specific supplement regimen that he outlines in his book. He is a huge advocate of Vitamin D and BCAA and advises all of his clients to incorporate them into their daily routines.

Vitamin D - This supplement is key to recovery and mental conditioning. Vitamin D keeps you going and your body full of energy.

BCAA – This supplement makes you feel more mobile (energetic) and helps with the rehabilitation process especially with respect to injury. BCAAs are highly recommended for faster recovery.

Dolvett prefers to eat foods that are all-natural and that you would find on an island such as: fruits, fish, grains, and veggies. He stays away from white foods (potatoes), packaged foods and always eats clean. One of his biggest tips is to stay on the outside aisle in the grocery store because that's where all of the healthier foods are. "When I eat I pretend I'm on an island and only have access to local food."

MENTAL STRATEGIES TO STAYING FIT

Dolvett meditates every day. His morning ritual is to stare into a flame and imagine a place of peace. When working with his clients (celebrities or otherwise) he tells them that meditation is the best practice before and after their workouts. "Some people say to stretch their muscles before and after workouts for the physical practice, but I subscribe to the mental aspect of working out so I have [them] stretch their minds before and after to be at peace." Dolvett believes that in order to be physically fit, you have to be mentally fit and strong like a warrior.

When it comes to recovery methods, he says "water, water, water!" Staying hydrated is a key element to his daily routine. "Remember you're on an island." He also incorporates essential fish oils for recovery gains as well as exercise bands and foam rollers for deep muscle stretches. Dolvett sticks mostly to dynamic stretching as most of his studio clients are clinically obese and need to wake up their muscles to begin with so he can get them on a regular routine that's right for them.

His final advice to anyone looking to spruce up their workouts is to mix it up once a week and try yoga, paddle boarding, biking, etc. "Shock your body in a new way. Working out should be fun and a major part of your life so it's important to get yourself out of a typical routine once in a while."

NOTES

CHAPTER EIGHT

WHAT'S NEXT?

Well, there you have it. We finally find ourselves at the end of this book because what I have to say on how to become a better, more elite athlete, and a better, more well-rounded person in life has already been tackled. So where do you go from here?

As you have read, it's inevitable that we all have areas we can improve—and I've provided various strategies for you to address these trouble spots in your life whether it be your nutrition, training, sleep, mental work, health care regimens and so on.

It is also evident that there is a lot of work that goes into living an "elite" life and being your best athlete. The key is to start somewhere (start anywhere… JUST START!) and begin working on improvement from there.

Personally, I like to make lists of all the things suggested in this book (and don't forget to check out the links and websites suggested) then I begin checking them off one by one. Then guess what? I repeat the entire process again. Yes, practice makes perfect.

Some of my favorite reminders:

Take BCAA during workout

Switch out protein powder and take 30 minutes post-workout

Block off 5 minutes a day for shoulder mobility

Spend 3 minutes in the morning looking over your goals

Everything in this book (all of the strategies, exercises, tips, tricks, tactics etc.) if followed the way I have outlined them WILL help you achieve your ultimate goals in your health and fitness and life in general. You may want to highlight them, jot them in a journal, or put them in your cell phone so you always have them close to you.

The key is getting them on a to-do list somewhere and sticking with your new plan to follow the Eliteness Movement that I have developed to help thousands of aspiring athletes and regular gym-goers to progress to in their lives.

Remember, I was once where you are—trying to learn all that you can about what it takes to become an elite person and athlete.

And what have I learned over all these years? I've learned that all of us were born and destined to become great and you can do it! But how many of us are tapping into our true potentials to do so?

Your journey to eliteness begins now… Good luck!!

NOTES

ABOUT
THE AUTHOR

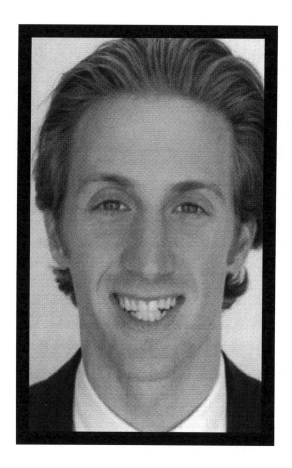

Dr. Austin Cohen is a sought-after and recognized health professional, athlete consultant, nutrition and fitness expert, and the Founder of Corrective Chiropractic, a thriving private chiropractic practice in Atlanta, Georgia. He is FMS Certified (Level 1 & 2) and has received post-doctorate training in structural care through Chiropractic Biophysics—and has done research on how healthy posture relates to optimal function, which has been published in the *Journal of Pediatric, Maternal & Family Health*. He is also a contributing author to the popular blog *Primal Docs* and has been featured on CNN, CBS, and The Weather Channel as an expert in his field.

Dr. Austin Cohen received his doctor of chiropractic degree from Life University in Atlanta, GA. He received his undergraduate training at Virginia Commonwealth University and received a Bachelor of Science in Biology. While pursuing his chiropractic studies, Dr. Cohen began focused studies on structural correction through the CBP and Pettibon protocol. He has always had a passion for serving families and helping people who could not get better through traditional and alternative means.

Dr. Cohen and his compassionate staff offer numerous services including Massage Therapy, Corrective Traction Exercises, Seminars and Workshops, Digital X-rays, and Digital Stress Scans and Muscle Scans—for a variety of clients ranging from pregnant women, children, and the active aging market; to weekend warriors and professional athletes, and those requiring rehabilitation for injury.

Dr. Cohen's professional and personal mission is to "lead, empower, and inspire my community to lead a proactive life through the principles of chiropractic." The uniqueness of his practice resides within Dr. Cohen's passion for helping people and wanting them to express 100% of their true potential. His dedication to his work with clients and professional athletes has proven over and over that people are capable of meeting their true expectations and becoming elite athletes if they so desire, or at the very least, are able to meet their own personal expectations they have set forth.

Dr. Cohen has made an incredible impact on the industry—particularly in how people achieve their mental and physical goals. His expertise in combining unique mobility strategies with proper health, fitness and supplementation modalities has enabled him to create and implement an "Eliteness Movement" which has changed the lives of people from all walks of life. Dr. Cohen does this by continuing to break down barriers and help people move beyond the capacity they think they are able to achieve at any given time. His insightful work is imperative to the future of health and wellness in America as we know it.

In his spare time, Dr. Cohen loves spending time with his wife, Shira, and beautiful one-year-old daughter, Harlow, as well as competing in CrossFit competitions and travelling to various places to observe animals in their natural habitat. His favorite place so far has been Victoria, Canada where one of his most memorable moments was watching orca whales swim in the wild.

WHAT PEOPLE ARE SAYING ABOUT DR. COHEN:

"I have worked with Dr. Cohen during my CrossFit competitions and his mentorship has always been a game changer in my performance. Once I receive an adjustment I can automatically feel the difference in my mobility and movement. Along with chiropractic services, Dr. Cohen has also suggested other tips and tricks to help me perform better and so far everything has worked." –Stacie Tovar

"Dr. Cohen began seeing me in the off-season when I left the Angels and began playing for the White Sox. I never saw a chiropractor regularly but Dr. Cohen helped with the rotation I had in my pelvis as well as clearing out my spine to get me performing better. When I come home to Atlanta during the off-season I always make it a point to see Dr. Cohen for chiropractic as well as his advice that he gives me during each adjustment." –Gordon Beckham

"I love everyone at Corrective Chiro! They are my very own 'get me patched up and put back together' team in Atlanta. As an athlete and trainer, I'm so thankful to have them on my side. I've recommended several people to Corrective Chiropractic for all services, and will continue to do so." -Lillian C

"Dr. Cohen was very affable and I'm very impressed by the diagnostic studies he conducted. It struck me he really wanted to determine the root of my problems and didn't just jump into providing adjustments, etc. without doing a thorough investigation. I'm looking forward to continued visits at CC." -Jonathan W

"Dr. Cohen is the best, and the entire team at CC is so knowledgeable and friendly, I just love this place. I look forward to my visits every week!" -Kristina G

"Dr. Cohen is one of the best chiropractors in Atlanta! He truly cares about his patients and is willing to address all areas of their health including nutrition. He also does free informative webinars, which are always on interesting topics. One of his staff members, Jessica, is a nutrition expert and often holds recipe nights and grocery store tours. I would recommend Dr. Cohen to my closest friends. Ever since seeing him over a year ago, I have had zero back pain." -Courtney H

"Dr. Cohen and his team are EXCELLENT! I have been a patient of his for two years now. I went to him with severe pain in my neck and later found out I had a bone spur. I could not even hold a purse on my shoulder or turn my head to the left while driving due to severe pain. I am now PAIN FREE and feel awesome." -Lisa T

For More Information and How You Can Reach Dr. Cohen:

Web: DrAustinCohen.com

Facebook: Facebook.com/draustincohen

Instagram: @draustincohen

Twitter: @atlantachiro

CORRECTIVE CHIROPRACTIC

2233 Peachtree Rd.

NE, Suite 204

Atlanta, GA 30309

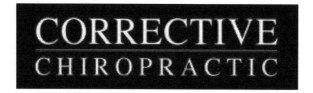

Made in the USA
Lexington, KY
04 May 2016